HerHormones

A Book for Men

Professor Shaughn O'Brien &
Dr Paula Briggs

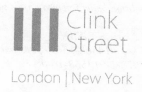

Clink
Street

London | New York

Published by Clink Street Publishing 2020

Copyright © 2020

First edition.

ISBN:
978-1-913568-15-3 - paperback
978-1-913568-16-0 - ebook

To all of the women who have been treated successfully and whose lives and relationships have been regained. And for the men who have understood...

Health Warning – Women are advised not to read this book

This book is exclusively for men. It concerns the influence of hormones on women and, importantly, all the secondary influences on men. Hormones are rather abstract, and cannot themselves be acknowledged, but their effects can be seen and experienced often without the association being recognised. Moreover, they can lead to an enormous impact on women's behavioural patterns, mood, physical appearance, self-worth, self-esteem, self-harm, relationships, aggressive acts and declining efficiency in work or at school environments. Significantly, hormones influence practically all aspects of women's conduct and behaviour and crucially, their quality of life. Certainly, this can have secondary detrimental influences on male partners, other family members and work contemporaries generally. Negative effects from hormones may go unrecognised for many years.

Avoidance of jargon is considered important in the descriptions in our book and where a medical word is demanded, it is explained. It is very much a book for men about women and, whilst we would discourage women from reading it, we do not discourage them from bringing it to the attention of their husbands, partners and sons.

Preface

Professor Shaughn O'Brien is Emeritus Professor of Obstetrics and Gynaecology of Keele University School of Medicine having been appointed Foundation Professor in 1989. His clinical post over that period of time was Consultant Obstetrician and Gynaecologist at Royal Stoke University Hospital. Prior to this he was Consultant at the Royal Free Hospital School of Medicine and Senior Lecturer at University of London. From 2004-7 he was Vice President of the Royal College of Obstetricians and Gynaecologists, chairman of the (now) British Society for Biopsychosocial Obstetrics and Gynaecology, chairman of the International Society for Premenstrual Disorders plus many more roles. For most of his career he undertook the whole spectrum of the specialty and developed clinical and research interests in disorders related to female hormones particularly PMS/PMDD, PCOS and the menopause.

Research interest: He is currently involved in research into the misdiagnosis of hormonal disorders which are inappropriately labelled psychiatric and he is Chief Coordinating Investigator of possibly the first drug ever to be developed specifically for PMDD. He retired from active clinical practice at the age of 71 to pursue a career in fine art, mainly sculpture, but at the transition felt it an opportunity to construct this book. Whilst there are many books on the topic of female hormones for the medical profession and for women, none has been written specifically for men.

Dr Paula Briggs is an Honorary Senior Lecturer at the University of Liverpool and a Consultant in Sexual & Reproductive Health at Liverpool Women's NHS Foundation

Trust. Prior to this she was a General Practitioner. She is a member of the Medical Advisory Council of the British Menopause Society.

She specialises in medical gynaecology including menopause management and premenstrual syndrome and is involved in research in this area of women's health. She is also currently involved in research into the misdiagnosis of hormonal disorders, which are inappropriately labelled as psychiatric conditions and follows Professor O'Brien as Chief Investigator of hopefully the first drug ever to be developed specifically for PMDD.

It was during the course of this clinical trial that they collaborated to share their expertise in relation to hormone disorders affecting women, but also men. This book is for men to help them understand and as a result will help men and women.

Contents

CHAPTER 1

Setting the scene

In men, hormones can be responsible for wars, murder, aggression and rape – and they make them smell! Female hormones have both obvious effects (physical sexual characteristics such as breast and genital development) and can also result in subtler changes. The less obvious changes affect vast numbers of people worldwide and every day – this is not widely recognised. Understanding female hormones is really important – it can save relationships, marriages and even lives. To most men, understanding female hormones might seem an impossible and daunting task. We hope that this book will help to make some if not all things clear, with a mixture of facts, real-life stories and a little speculation.

Hormonal effects are complicated. One hormone often acts with another – or more often more than one other. The effects of hormones can be different at different times depending on which cell, tissue or body organ the hormone is affecting. The actions of hormones change throughout the month from puberty, during pregnancies and after the menopause – indeed throughout life. There are effects on the fetus in the womb, during childhood; before, during and after puberty; over the course of a month through the menstrual cycle; and throughout pregnancy. There are complex effects leading up to the menopause and beyond. This describes *normal* hormonal processes. On top of this, some women experience problems associated with *abnormal* responses to normal hormone cycles such as in premenstrual syndrome. Finally, we must also consider the reasons for benefits and side effects of hormones that women are prescribed, either for illnesses or for potential benefits, such as HRT (hormone replacement therapy), subfertility treatment or contraception.

A BIT ABOUT HORMONES GENERALLY

There are many different hormones. The first to be discovered was insulin, which is associated with diabetes. Diabetes is due to insulin deficiency/resistance and can be type 1 or type 2. Another well-known hormone is thyroid hormone.

Naturally produced hormones are made in the body and released from glands called endocrine glands. They make their way in the bloodstream to other parts of the body, where they then have specific actions, which, as we have said, can be different at different places in the body, different ages and times – and the effects of the same hormone can be different between the sexes.

We have all heard of steroid hormones in the controversial area of sport performance enhancement and bodybuilding. But steroids are only one of many groups of hormones. There are many hormones and there are many steroids; anabolic steroids are those used by bodybuilders (male and female) and possibly some athletes to "improve" appearance or performance. Other steroids, corticosteroids, are used to prevent inflammation and are used in disorders such as inflammation of the lungs as in asthma or of the joints in arthritis. The moon-faced appearance of patients following prolonged use of oral corticosteroids is reasonably well known. Other steroids are the so-called "sex" steroids. These sound more interesting (!) and the remainder of this book deals with this area. The names are well known to all of us because they affect everyone irrespective of gender. Testosterone is classically recognised as a male hormone, although it is also an important female hormone. Oestrogen is the hormone normally associated with women. Progesterone is also extremely important and we will come back to this in detail throughout the book. There are other sex steroids that occur naturally in the body and many others that are manufactured by the pharmaceutical industry.

This book concentrates on how the sex steroids work in the human female. It looks at their physical and psychological effects, how they occur, how they go wrong and, if they do go wrong what and how treatment can be provided. We have seen partners of patients who treat their wives like a commodity. They take their wife to the gynaecologist and say that "she" is no longer functioning the same way as when they first got her. Fix it! Nothing is said quite as blatantly as this, but this is the underlying attitude. It denotes extreme lack of sensitivity and respect for their partner and a complete lack of understanding of the subtle effects of hormones within the female body – not just the physical effects but perhaps more importantly the psychological and emotional factors. We hope that this book will lead to a better understanding of the reasons for changes in women, to help men to develop their understanding and show them how to work with their partners to overcome what can be very major issues in a relationship.

By focusing on the sex steroids – oestrogen, progesterone and testosterone (yes women produce a lot of testosterone) – the whole issue will be simplified.

So let's start with the basics and look at a few names and what they mean. You may need to refer back to these throughout your reading, so it might be useful to put a marker in these pages.

A **hormone** is a chemical messenger. Hormones are produced (or secreted) by one cell or tissue and moved to another through the bloodstream, unless the target tissue is close by. Some hormones are produced all the time. Others occur intermittently, in cycles, during pregnancy or in short regular pulses. Levels may change through the day, months or year.

To be effective hormones have a specific structural (molecular) shape and they fit into a receptor of complimentary shape – exactly like a lock and a key, the hormone being the key, the receptor being the lock.

Sex hormones

Just to recap, different hormones and receptors have different structures (in the same way as a key will only open one specific lock). Some hormones are made up of a few amino acids, called peptides. Amino acids are the building blocks (bricks) of peptides (walls), polypeptides (rooms) and proteins (houses). A few amino acids joined are peptides; more are polypeptides and a large number of peptides are proteins. Many hormones are peptides, polypeptides and proteins. Steroids and sex steroid hormones are made of carbon rings, with different bits and pieces of, nitrogen, oxygen and hydrogen molecules added. Very slight differences in the added bits can give extremely different actions. All of these sex steroids are built from cholesterol. More on all of this later...

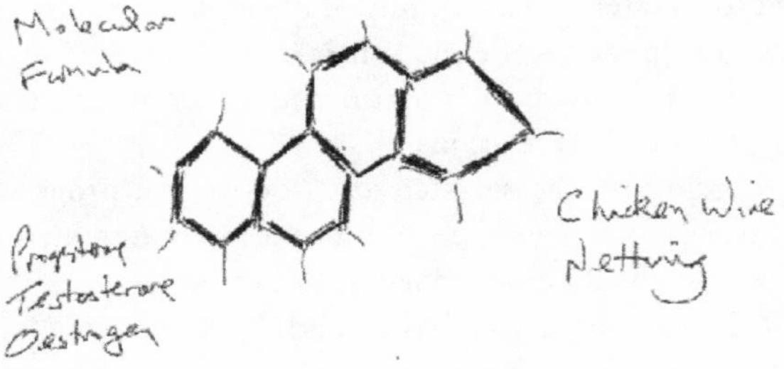

Figure 1

Molecular Structure of Sex Steroids

The sex hormones oestrogen, progesterone and testosterone have surprisingly similar structures with very small chemical substitutions having a major change in their effects.

The molecule greatly magnified looks like chicken wire netting.

Some well-known hormones

Insulin (protein): if this is lacking it gives rise to (type 1) diabetes

Thyroid (peptide): ihe thyroid gland can be overactive or underactive

Cortisol (steroid): controls many things including inflammation

Progesterone (sex steroid): produced by the ovary in the second half of the menstrual cycle

Oestrogen (sex steroid): produced by the ovary most of the time; stops being produced after the menopause

Testosterone (sex steroid): produced by men in the testes and women in the ovary and by both men and women in the adrenal gland – it is responsible (with many other environmental and biopsychosocial factors) for male and female sex drive.

There are many terms which are useful to know when thinking, talking and reading about hormones and the following list may be of use.

Endocrine means anything to do with hormones. An **endocrinologist** is a doctor who diagnoses and treats people with endocrine problems and a **gynaecological endocrinologist** is a gynaecologist whose main interest is the hormonal aspects of women's health – the focus of this book – these are the expert areas of the authors.

Endocrine glands are found throughout the body. They produce hormones. The ovaries and testes are the female and male endocrine glands.

There are two **ovaries** (each called an **ovary**). These are the main female organs and they lie protected in the pelvis by the pelvic bones. They produce an egg each month (for fertilisation) – this is a single cell initially and nothing like a chicken's egg; they produce the female hormones (sex steroids) oestrogen, progesterone and also testosterone.

The **pituitary gland** is another endocrine organ, which is very important in relation to women's hormones and menstrual cycles. It lies in the middle of the head, behind the eyes. It produces hormones that send signals to other endocrine glands – it controls the ovary to produce its hormones. Quite complex, but Chapter 4 will unravel the details in a "sex steroid hormones for dummies" kind of way (apologies to those who already know some of this).

The **hypothalamus** is the part of the brain immediately above the pituitary gland. This produces very small hormones, which drive the pituitary gland.

More of this later as well…

The HPO axis is actually the hypothalamo-pituitary-ovarian axis. It's worth knowing this. It sounds and is rather complicated but, to simplify, it is the pathway where the hormones from the brain connect to the ovary to produce the menstrual cycle pre-menopause. All will be revealed in later chapters…

Hormone receptor – Hormone activity is complex, but to understand their disorders and their treatment it is enough to realise that they operate on a lock and key principle. The hormone is the key and has a specific shape. As it passes around the bloodstream it tries various locks until it finds one that fits. When it does, this turns on a series of chemical activities which give rise to that hormone's actions.

Puberty is when the sex hormones start up.

Menarche is when periods start.

Menstruation or the 'menstrual **period**' is the bleeding associated with each cycle. It normally lasts three to six days.

A **menstrual cycle** is usually about 28 days and is the time from day 1 of a period until the next period starts.

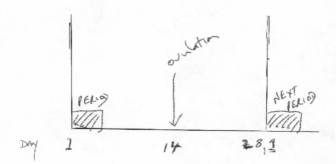

Figure 2

The days of the menstrual cycle showing the first period and a second period 28 days later.

Release of the egg [ovulation] happens on about the 14th day of this cycle.

The period length can vary but will be about 3-6 days in most women.

Day of the menstrual cycle – Every day during the menstrual cycle is given a number. The first day of the last menstrual period is day 1. So the period starts on day one and ovulation occurs on about day 14 (halfway through) with the last day of the cycle (before the next period begins) being day 28 (in a regular 28-day cycle). Ovulation occurs 14 days before the beginning of a normal period, unless fertilisation and pregnancy occur. The normal range of cycle length is 23–35 days, between the first day of one period and the next with many women having periods outside this range. For instance, when ovulation occurs infrequently, the timing of the cycle is lost and the time between periods can be very long – we will see later how this happens in women with PCOS (polycystic ovary syndrome) in chapter 9.

LMP – the last menstrual period – This is the first day of the last menstrual period. It is the one piece of information that should always be asked of women if trying to work out matters related to the cycle (pregnancy/abnormal bleeding/perimenopause).

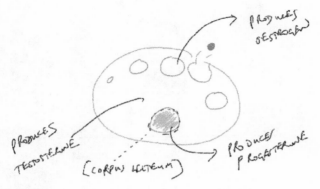

Figure 3

In the first half of the cycle the follicle – a cyst-like structure –
produces oestrogen. After ovulation when the egg (red dot) is released,
the follicle becomes the yellow body [corpus luteum]. The yellow is
cholesterol from which the sex steroids are made.

This produces progesterone mainly and oestrogen. Other parts of the
ovary produce testosterone.

Ovulation is when the ovary releases its egg (ovum), normally
on day 14 of the cycle, if the woman has a regular 28-day cycle.
After this, the ovary produces the hormone progesterone,
the level of which peaks about seven days before the start of
the next period (menstrual bleeding). The egg in the ovary is
contained in a little sack called a **follicle** – the follicle produces
only oestrogen. After the egg has been released, the follicle turns
into a **corpus luteum**, which produces not only oestrogen but
a large amount of progesterone as well.

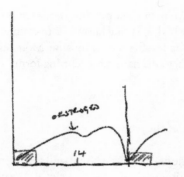

Figure 4

The pattern of oestrogen production by the ovarian follicle and corpus luteum throughout both halves of the menstrual cycle.

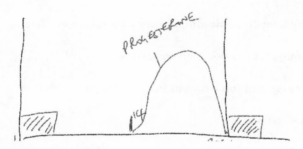

Figure 5

The pattern of progesterone production from the corpus lutum is confined mainly to the second half of the cycle.

This term comes from Latin meaning yellow body – it is yellow as it contains cholesterol and as we have said earlier cholesterol is the chemical from which sex steroids are made.

Menopause is when the periods finally stop. This is not really a problem in itself, but the periods stop because the hormones are first changing and then ceasing altogether, which can cause many problems.

HRT is **hormone replacement therapy**. This treatment puts back a synthetic version of the body's natural hormones to counteract the effects of the lack of hormones after the menopause. Most oestrogen given in HRT is identical to the naturally occurring form.

The **endometrium** is the lining of the womb.

The **uterus** is the same as the womb.

There will some conditions or disorders that will keep cropping up. An initial introduction to them may be helpful. We will not use the more complicated terms very often and actually most modern doctors and gynaecologists now do the same.

Period problems [medical term in brackets]:

Heavy menstrual bleeding, heavy periods [menorrhagia]

Too frequent periods [polymenorrhoea]

Too heavy and too frequent Periods [polymenorrhagia]

Prolonged periods

Absent periods [amenorrhoea]

Painful Periods [dysmenorrhoea]

Intermenstrual bleeding [bleeding between periods]

Lining of the womb – [endometrium]

Endometriosis is a condition where tissue of the lining the womb (endometrium) grows in various parts of the pelvis and elsewhere, places that it should not be. This can lead to pain and fertility problems.

Subfertility: many books have been written on this problem. The cause may be something in the male system, in the female system or in both partners. If it is in the female, then it may be mechanical (such as a blockage of the tubes) or it may be hormonal (perhaps she is not ovulating).

Fibroids: the normal uterus is made of muscle. Sometimes the fibre and muscle are formed into fibrous/muscular balls. These can be quite large, e.g. the size of a cricket ball and sometimes bigger. It is the position rather than the size of fibroids which causes problems such as heavy bleeding, difficulty conceiving or pressure. Fibroids are nearly always benign (not cancer); they only very rarely become cancerous.

Polycystic ovaries (PCO), polycystic ovary syndrome (PCOS): PCO is just a type of ovary affecting about a fifth of women and is not a problem. PCOS is one of the most difficult conditions to understand. It has a wide range of effects. Essentially, the hormone cycle and the normal monthly release of eggs goes wrong. Hormones are mixed up and eggs are not released regularly. This subject needs a whole chapter (see Chapter 9).

Bio-identical hormones, The concept of bio-identical hormones has been introduced in recent years and may be a marketing ploy by "specialist pharmacies". There is a small summary explaining what this means in the HRT section of this book (Chapter 12).

That is enough on definitions and terms for the moment.

HerHormones

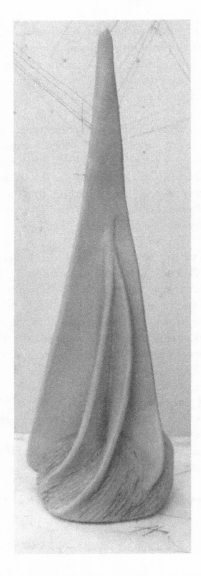

The Shard Temple of Gender Equality 2019

CHAPTER 2

A basic guide to female anatomy

Let's start from the top. The brain is an organ that is different in men than it is in women. It is probably different in many ways right from the beginning of life. Apart from local neurotransmitters it does not really produce hormones but it does respond to them in a big way.

In the middle of the brain is the hypothalamus, which sits just above the pituitary gland. The pituitary has two parts: one part secretes hormones and the other part stores and releases hormones in response to chemical messages that it receives from the hypothalamus. The hypothalamus has a blood supply linked to the pituitary, so that it can send chemical messages to it. Once it gets the messages, the pituitary sends its own chemical messages to the ovaries. This is what stimulates the ovarian hormone cycle.

THE HORMONES PRODUCED BY THE PITUITARY GLAND
In the context of female hormone cycles, there are two important hormones produced by the pituitary gland:

1. FSH – follicle stimulating hormone. Not surprisingly this stimulates the the follicles, one of which becomes the "dominant" follicle to develop and to produce oestrogen and also ovum or "the egg".

2. LH – luteinising hormone. After ovulation, this turns the follicle into a "corpus luteum" or "yellow body", which produces the hormone progesterone in the second half of the cycle from the cholesterol, which has a yellow colour and hence the Latin name (luteum). LH is actually responsible for ovulation and would be better described as OH or ovulating hormone! When the endometrium is well-prepared for the arrival of the fertilised egg and the egg itself in the follicle is "ripe" there is a surge (the LH/OH surge) lasting less than a day which makes ovulation happen.

THE PELVIS

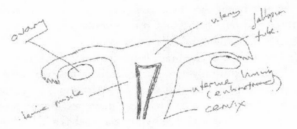

Figure 6

The anatomy of the normal female pelvis showing the uterus and cervix leading into the top of the vagina.

Also shown are the two ovaries and the two fallopian tubes.

The pelvis is the area of the body below the abdomen (belly button level) and above the legs. The soft parts inside are surrounded/protected by the bony part of the pelvis. Inside this protective "shell" of the pelvic skeleton, there are muscles, joints, bladder, bowel, womb, ovaries, tubes, nerves and more. Forget those – apart from the fact that they are close together and when there is pelvic pain it is often hard to be sure which one is responsible for the pain.

The important organs for this book are the uterus (womb), the tubes (fallopian tubes) the ovaries (ovaries) and the brain. There are two fallopian tubes, two ovaries and one uterus. Actually, when these pelvic organs were developing they were formed from two tubes; the lower part fused to make one organ, the uterus, while the fallopian tubes remained separate. We do not really need to dwell on the tubes, which transport eggs and sperms for fertilisation. They are not of interest in our current context with the focus mainly on the effect of hormones on women and indirectly men, though infection in the tubes can cause pain and fertility problems.

However, the ovaries are all-important in relation to female hormones. Hormones affect bleeding (from the lining of the womb) and therefore the ovaries and uterus are central to everything to come in the rest of this book.

Just to prepare the ground for what comes later, we should say that the lining of the womb builds up under the influence of oestrogen. This hormone is the main player before ovulation; following ovulation (middle of the cycle), progesterone is the main player throughout the second half of the menstrual cycle. It prevents the lining of the womb becoming too thick – in fact a woman's own progesterone or prescribed synthetic progestogens can prevent cancer of the lining of the womb by preventing continued proliferation.

The ovaries are buried deep in the pelvis for protection – not like the testicles! They are about 3.5 x 2.5 x 2cm. They are white and wrinkled in young menstruating women and are small and smooth before puberty and shrink and become smooth again after the menopause – the opposite to skin! The normal ovary can have different appearances at different times of the monthly cycle. First there are little "cysts" – one of these contains "the egg" which will be released at ovulation. When ovulation occurs, it ruptures from the surface of the ovary releasing the egg and fluid. Once ovulation has occurred, this cyst becomes a yellow blob or "yellow body" (in Latin – "corpus luteum"). As already mentioned it is yellow because it contains lots of cholesterol – sex steroids are produced from cholesterol. It is converted into the hormone progesterone, which is released into the body from the time of ovulation until the period starts.

The uterus is shaped like an upside-down pear with the stalk taken out; the dimple where the stalk would be being the cervix and this is where cervical smears tests are taken from (a sample of the cells). Cut it in half lengthways the uterus looks more like an avocado with the stone removed. The main part of the uterus is made almost entirely of muscle. In the middle is a flattened space. Around this space is the lining of the uterus, called the endometrium. This lining builds up to a nice thick bed every month, just in case a fertilised egg comes along. If there is no pregnancy, then hormone levels fall and the lining breaks down – i.e. a period. If there is no baby to grow, the lining is shed from the wall of the uterus and the blood and other stuff passes from the cavity through the narrow canal in the cervix to the vagina. Mostly tampons or sanitary pads keep this all invisible.

The visible (external) parts of the female reproductive or genital tract are more familiar territory. They also respond to the hormones described above. The vagina needs oestrogen to stay healthy and lubricated. After the menopause (when oestrogen is no longer produced by the ovaries) the lining (skin) of the vagina becomes thin, smooth, sensitive and easily damaged by trauma and friction. This can be a serious problem for a couple as sex can be painful or impossible. It can usually be very easily sorted out, but women (and men) often suffer in silence for years. The clitoris, labia and vulva also depend on oestrogen. The G spot is not a physical entity – well, one research paper claims to have identified a physical structure. Rumour has it that the G spot was invented by feminists when men discovered where the clitoris was, in order to keep them guessing!

Above are terms that will be repeated most often throughout the book.

Professor Shaughn O'Brien & Dr Paula Briggs

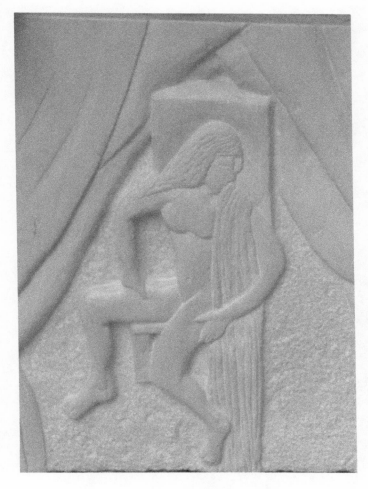

Seated Nude 2015

CHAPTER 3

What the ovaries do each month and throughout life

This is a highly complex subject and if you do not understand it then you may not understand the rest of the book. You must understand the cycle of the ovaries and it would be better if you understood the HPO axis as well. What follows, we hope, is a relatively simple explanation of the hormone cycle of the ovary. We use it as a background for patients before explaining their gynaecological problems. It is also the way we teach medical students on their gynaecology attachment.

Do not read on until you understand it!

While still in the womb, in the early stages of her mother's pregnancy, a female fetus has three million eggs in her ovaries. By the time she is born, only 750,000 remain and by puberty, this number has gone down to 250,000. Not all of these eggs are needed. Between puberty and the menopause about 40 years, there are no more than 13 ovulations each year. So, the maximum number of eggs actually needed for ovulation is about 480. However, many more than one egg begins to develop in each cycle. The biggest one – the dominant egg/dominant follicle is released and the others are reabsorbed, so the supply is used up more rapidly. Pregnancy slows this process down, as ovulation stops (for obvious reasons). Eggs are also prevented from developing when a woman is taking certain types of contraception, especially the combined pill. There are also some gynaecological disorders where there is no ovulation. Generally speaking, then, ovulation occurs once a month from puberty around age 11 to 13, but sometimes later, and continues up to the menopause, around age 51 (normal range 45 to 55).

Many people think that interfering with ovulation is unnatural. In truth, it is menstruation that is unnatural! One hundred years ago, young girls began their periods at 12 or 13, had started ovulating regularly by 15, were married by 17, had eight pregnancies, six of which survived, breastfed between and died at the age of the menopause. So, no contraception, no periods, no dysmenorrhoea, no PMS, less ovarian cancer, no endometriosis, possibly less uterine cancer, with only one partner less cervical cancer, maybe less breast cancer and no menopause and no postmenopausal problems. A depressing picture? Possibly, but one that reflects a much more naturally biological life pattern for the human female than today's long life with many menstrual cycles.

So, several eggs begin to develop each month. Each one is a tiny sack-like structure or follicle and usually only one becomes the main one, the dominant follicle. This has two functions – it contains the egg (ovum) and also the cells that are capable of producing hormones. These cells produce the sex steroid oestrogen, in ever-increasing amounts. The follicle grows during this time to become just over 20 millimetres in diameter. At this point in time, the hormone levels are at their best for ovulation and the egg is desperate to come out of the follicle to "mate" with the sperm or to undergo fertilisation and produce the beginnings of a new baby. If this happens, a huge change in hormones will occur. But, if pregnancy does not occur (which is more frequent) then a normal menstrual cycle results. First, the follicle, which previously contained the ovum and produced oestrogen, now starts to produce not only oestrogen, but large amounts of another hormone, progesterone. It is no longer called a follicle, and is now the corpus luteum.

These two hormones, oestrogen and progesterone, prepare the lining of the womb for a potential pregnancy to embed and develop. If no pregnancy occurs, there is no need for a lining (bed), so the corpus luteum stops working and the two hormone levels fall. There is nothing to keep the lining of the womb ready to nurture a pregnancy any longer, so it is shed from the womb as a menstrual period. A period will last around five days in most women. It is not just the lining of the womb that is shed, but blood and other secretions as well.

WHAT DOES THE UTERUS DO EACH MONTH?

The womb does not do anything unless it is told to – just the opposite of teenagers who will not do anything they are told, and if you tell them to do something, they will do it less!

We are on Chapter 3 now – advanced grade! – may we drop the term womb and say uterus? And drop the term womb lining and say endometrium? More often than not the uterus does as it is told by the hormones produced by the ovary. As we saw earlier, the main parts of the uterus are the muscular body, the cervix, which is at the top of the vagina and the uterine lining, the endometrium. The body of the uterus, the cervix (and the mucus in the cervix) do change through the cycle but the only important changes for us to consider are those occurring in the endometrium.

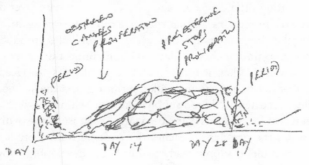

Figure 7

The normal cyclical changes of the lining of the womb [endometrium] throughout the cycle.

On day one the tissue collapses and this is the onset of the period.

Oestrogen from the ovary stimulates it to grow and *proliferate*.

Progesterone stops it proliferating.

It also creates changes in the endometrium making it welcoming and feeding an arriving fertilised egg should there be one. So progesterone makes it *secretory*.

33

Through the month the endometrium has three phases.

1. Menstruation: the phase where menstrual bleeding ("the period") occurs. This happens when the hormone levels of the previous cycle fall, because fertilisation and pregnancy didn't happen.

In the first half of the cycle, also called the follicular or proliferative phase, the endometrium thickens waiting for the arrival of the fertilised egg. Oestrogen produced by the developing follicles in the ovary, before the dominant follicle is chosen prior to ovulation, command the uterus to make the lining thicken in preparation for a possible pregnancy.

In the second half of the cycle, also called the luteal or secretory phase following ovulation, progesterone from the ovary (a) produces secretions to "feed" the new pregnancy and (b) prevents proliferation (overgrowth) and also prevents cancer.

So, the period occurs when there is no pregnancy.

Remember the corpus luteum, which forms after ovulation and produces the hormone progesterone? Without a pregnancy this collapses and nearly all the endometrium is shed and passes through the cervix as "the period". A thin base layer of endometrium remains, so that the cycle can start over again.

At the beginning of the cycle the follicles produce oestrogen again which stimulates the remaining thin layer of endometrium. When it is stimulated it proliferates. To recap, what this means is that the endometrium grows thicker and develops an extensive blood supply. The idea behind this is that when it is at its peak this coincides with the release of the ovum and when the pregnancy reaches the endometrium there is a really good blood supply ready to "feed" the developing baby. So, proliferation occurs because of oestrogen.

In fact, if there was only oestrogen then the endometrium would continue to grow and proliferate, so much so that cancer could potentially occur. Most of the time, this does not happen, because progesterone stops proliferation and actually controls the growth of the endometrium. It also provides the clock for the timing of the cycle, resulting in a regular period when fertilisation and implantation (pregnancy) do not occur.

Remember, after ovulation, the corpus luteum produces large amounts of progesterone which balances the effect of oestrogen prior to ovulation. Progesterone also provides glycogen (a high-energy carbohydrate), "food" for a new pregnancy, should that occur.

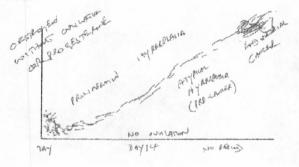

Figure 8

Effect on Endometrium showing what happens if ovulation does not occur and there is no progesterone. The cells proliferate further, the endometrium becoming thicker, overactive, atypical, abnormal, ultimately leading to the risk of endometrial cancer.

So there are two phases of the cycle and they both have two names!!

The first half of the cycle is called the follicular phase (because there is a follicle in the ovary) or the proliferative phase (because the endometrium is proliferating). The second half is called the luteal phase (because the ovary has the corpus luteum) or the secretory phase (because the endometrium is 'secreting').

HerHormones

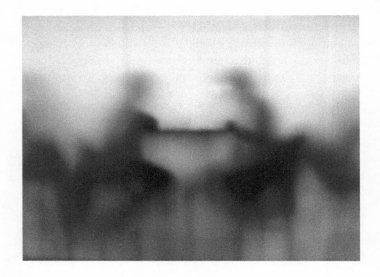

Important to Talk 2019

CHAPTER 4

What do the hormones produced by the ovaries do throughout the body?

This will be answered in detail in subsequent chapters in relation to specific hormonal problems. These include common conditions such as heavy periods, menopause related symptoms and pre-menstrual syndrome (PMS).

This is a short chapter as we thought you needed a break from the intensity of the first three chapters!

There are few places in the human body that are not affected by hormones and this is particularly true for sex hormones. Bone, brain, blood vessels, blood, joints, bladder, bowel, kidneys, breasts, uterus, vagina and eyes – the list is almost endless.

We know that from studying what happens when there is no oestrogen, that oestrogen is important for women. There is no oestrogen after the menopause, when the ovaries have been removed at operation or when certain drugs are given to induce a temporary menopause. Also, of course, there is no oestrogen before puberty, but that lack of oestrogen does not have the same effect.Now have a break, a beer even!

More later!

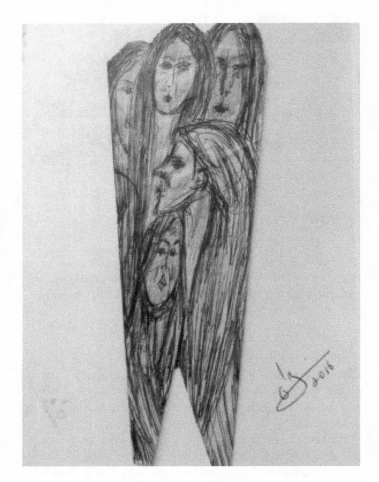

Not Alone 2016

CHAPTER 5

Treatments which affect hormone cycles and menstruation

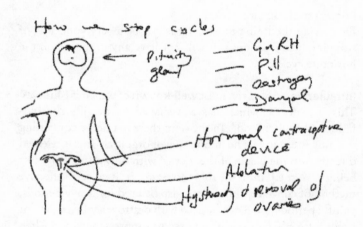

Figure 9

How we stop hormone cycles. It is well known that, at the menopause the hormones cycle stops and all the menstrual cycle problems disappear.

But until that happens all of the problems described may need treating.

Stopping the hormone cycles is one way in seriously affected patients – it will often help. Details are in the text but here is a summary list.

SURGERY

Hysterectomy
This procedure removes the uterus and normally the cervix. Hormone cycles will continue, but there is no longer any bleeding.

Removal of Ovaries
This is called bilateral oophorectomy. This procedure removes the hormone cycles and the uterus and fallopian tubes are often removed at the same time when the procedure is called hysterectomy and bilateral salpingo-oophorectomy – in effect, it will produce a premature *surgical* menopause.

Endometrial Ablation
Destroying the lining of the uterus can be a very good way of stopping heavy periods – it will not have any influence on the hormone cycles.

Intrauterine system, the most well-known of which is Mirena®
This is a device which has a T-shaped frame like the old-fashioned copper "coil". In the stem there is a sleeve containing the progesterone-like hormone – levonorgestrel. This is released directly into the inside of the uterus, with only a small amount being absorbed into the bloodstream. It is a very effective method of contraception. It can also be used for heavy periods, painful periods and it can be used with oestrogen when a patient needs it for HRT or it is being used to suppress ovulation when treating PMS.

MEDICAL

Hormonal

GnRH Analogues
These drugs are very useful – they block the function of the

pituitary gland and so shut down the hormone production and hormone cycles. In men they are used to shut down the production of testosterone to treat prostate cancer. In women they can be used for endometriosis, PMS, heavy periods, painful periods and shrinking fibroids, usually prior to surgery. They are also used in the treatment of subfertility. They can be given daily, inhaled through the nose or by depot injection for one or three months.

FSH and LH

These are the synthetic versions of the pituitary hormones and are given to women not ovulating, as part of fertility treatment, especially where lots of eggs are required for IVF. We are not discussing subfertility in this book.

HRT

Hormone cycles can be recreated after a natural or premature menopause by using the two hormones of the menstrual cycle, oestrogen and progesterone. A whole chapter is dedicated to this topic.

Oral Contraception

The combined pill is a whole book topic in itself. Its main action is to stop ovulation by suppressing the hypothalamus and pituitary gland. Of course, because it is formulated using both oestrogen and progestogen (progesterone-like hormones), there will be many peripheral hormonal effects both positive and negative. There will still be bleeding unless used continuously without taking the seven-day break. Non-contraceptive benefits associated with combined pills include the management of endometriosis, heavy periods, painful periods, PMS, polycystic ovary syndrome and acne.

Progestogens

This is the term usually used to mean artificial or synthetic progesterone-like hormone therapies. They are used for many purposes, again including endometriosis, heavy periods, PMS (though as we will see they can sometimes also cause PMS-type symptoms), PCOS, and as part of HRT. They are used alone for contraception in the progestogen-only pill, injection, implant and Mirena ® when it is necessary to avoid oestrogen therapy or by choice.

Non-hormonal
Antifibrinolytics and Non-steroidal anti-inflammatory drugs

These drugs reduce blood loss (from the uterus in women with heavy periods and in nosebleeds!). They have a direct action on coagulation processes and will be discussed again in the next chapter on heavy menstrual bleeding (heavy periods).

Professor Shaughn O'Brien & Dr Paula Briggs

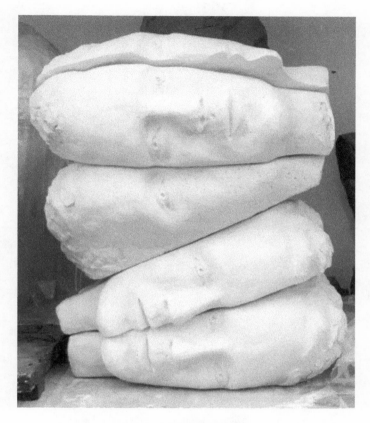

The Challenges for Men 2019

CHAPTER 6

Menstrual Problems

We are afraid we have to talk about menstrual bleeding at some stage. We have already seen that the hormones, oestrogen and progesterone, control the lining of the uterus, preparing for possible pregnancy, then shedding if this does not occur. Along with the blood there are secretions and cells. We have seen that the "perfect period", if there is such a thing, lasts about five days – in a "perfect cycle" there are 28 days from the beginning of one period to the start of the next. Total blood loss in a "perfect period" is about 30–45 millilitres. Many women will attend their GP with an abnormality or at least a change in periods at some time in their life. If you go back to the list of definitions (Chapter 1 and 2) you can see that there are quite a few changes that can occur. Let's talk about them briefly and see which ones should give cause for concern and which are merely a nuisance. We will finish by talking about everything you need to know about heavy periods. No periods: Waiting for periods to begin can cause anxiety for young girls (and more so their parents). There is a desire for normality and having periods signifies sexual maturity. Adolescence is a time of high hormone levels and keeping up with the competition is important from a biopsychosocial perspective. The time they start varies between age 12–14 but 10–16 is not uncommon. If they have not occurred by 15 or 16, then a visit to the GP may be sensible if only for reassurance. If they have not begun by 17, then investigations should be undertaken, even though there are late developers who have no problems. There are a vast number of potential causes of what is known in medical terms as primary amenorrhoea and we do not intend to go into these in great depth. The problems can be mechanical (for example a blocked vagina due to an imperforate hymen), hormonal (delayed or absent hormones), genetic and chromosomal (missing female X chromosome). The presence or absence of secondary sexual characteristics (pubic and axillary hair and breast development) will help define the possible causes of amenorrhoea (no periods). Significant problems are relatively rare and so reassurance is the usual outcome.

This is not the book to go into detail as it aims to deal with the more common problems – suffice to say, any delay in commencing bleeding should be discussed with the GP for possible referral to a general or paediatric/adolescent gynaecologist. Unfortunately, the commonest cause of no periods is pregnancy. Young women are highly fertile and pregnancy is possible even from first ovulation, which predates menstruation.

HEAVY PERIODS

Most women will go through a phase of heavy periods at some time in their life. It can be painful, distressing, embarrassing, and affects general health and wellbeing. It is distressing because the affected woman may believe she has cancer. It can be embarrassing because of accidents – blood in the bed, on clothes, on seats; it can stop women going out at all and can interfere with work. Often heavy periods are painful, sometimes very painful. If there is sufficient bleeding then anaemia can occur giving rise to tiredness, feeling faint or dizzy, shortness of breath and weakness.

THE CAUSES

There are many causes:

Hormonal causes

Failure to ovulate is the commonest reason for heavy bleeding. The lining of the uterus becomes too thick and sheds chaotically. This is common at extremes of reproductive life, menarche when periods start, and in the perimenopause.

In simple terms, no ovulation = no progesterone = oestrogen only cycles = build-up of the uterine lining and no regular menstrual clock. If this goes to an extreme level, the lining can become overactive (endometrial hyperplasia) which increases the risk of cancer (endometrial adenocarcinoma). This is not that common of course, but is one of the reasons why a woman with heavy periods may need a biopsy or hysteroscopy (camera). We have always said that any woman with abnormal bleeding over the age of 40 needs to be properly investigated. The recent NICE guidance suggests over 45. Cancer of the womb is not common, but is becoming commoner. Obesity is a risk factor and unfortunately this is becoming more common. Other risk factors include not having had children, polycystic ovary syndrome, diabetes and hypertension.

Underactive thyroid (hypothyroidism) is another cause of heavy periods– do not ask how this works as we do not think anyone knows! It can easily be treated by replacing thyroxine in tablet form. Routine investigation of heavy periods does not necessitate checking thyroid hormone levels in the blood, but this is sometimes done when there are other symptoms suggestive of hypothyroidism.

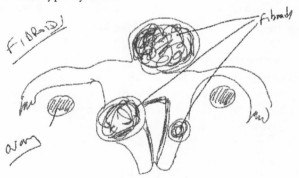

Figure 10

Fibroids are common. They are balls of muscle from the uterine wall. They can be located in different parts of the uterine wall and cause a variety of problems but particularly heavy periods.

Fibroids

The uterus is made of muscle. Sometimes the muscle comes together with fibrous tissue to form balls/fibroids. The size of fibroids is very variable, but they can be quite large, e.g. the size of a cricket ball. They are nearly always benign (not cancer) and very rarely become cancerous. Since ultrasound scans have become so detailed it seems as if nearly every woman has at least one small fibroid! Once identified they can cause anxiety although there is rarely a need to worry. The position is more important than the size in relation to heavy bleeding. Fibroids on the inside of the womb change the shape of the cavity and the surface area that women bleed from. Multiple fibroids, even small ones make the uterus bulky, again increasing the surface area from which a woman bleeds.

Polyps

These are also benign, common and can lead to heavy periods or bleeding between the periods. Bleeding between the periods nearly always needs gynaecological investigation although structural causes are less common than ovulatory dysfunction – the menstrual cycle going wrong! Polyps may result in the woman having a hysteroscopy (see below) when the polyps can be removed in a straightforward fashion.

Endometriosis

Endometriosis is commonly associated with heavy periods. There are many different ways that this can be treated and a whole section (below) is dedicated to this condition and its treatment.

Bleeding disorders

The bleeding disorder that you will likely have heard of is haemophilia. This occurs in boys and men, but is genetically transmitted by the mother. The mother is not usually affected, but there can be low levels of the coagulation factor, factor VIII, in carrier females. Other bleeding disorders which do occur in females are similar, such as Christmas disease (which actually causes problems all year round!) and von Willebrand's disease. They all affect the clotting mechanisms and so what should be the normal menstrual bleed becomes problematic. If detected, then women should be cared for by a haematologist with a gynaecologist taking over if the bleeding cannot be managed by a haematologist alone.

Don't Know

There are many conditions in the medical world where the underlying cause has not yet been identified. Rather than admit that they do not know something, doctors call this idiopathic. Actually this means they do not know, but they know that they do not know! For heavy menstrual bleeding the term dysfunctional uterine bleeding has been used for many years. It means that anatomical pathological causes have been excluded such as fibroids and polyps and that the cause is not related to a structural abnormality. It is most likely that the cause has got something to do with hormones!! In addition, coagulation of menstrual blood is likely to be influenced by a group of chemicals called prostaglandins which affect closure of the blood vessels at the base of the endometrial lining. Just briefly on prostaglandins, as it will help the understanding of one of the methods of treatment: These are very small, locally active chemicals, which are produced in many sites. Of relevance here, are those in the lining and muscle wall of the uterus. They can affect muscle contraction and blood vessel closure. They cause pain because of contractions. They are the same prostaglandins that are used in obstetrics to produce contractions of the uterine muscle to begin labour! When they are released during a period, they cause characteristic period pain. If we block their production with drugs (non-steroidal anti-inflammatory drugs such as ibuprofen and mefenamic acid) pain and bleeding can be reduced.

Treatment of Heavy Periods

Often, women do not need any treatment medical or surgical. If they do, this can be with medication (drugs), which:

- affect the prostaglandins controlling the bleeding from blood vessels (non-steroidals) or the coagulation mechanisms (antifibrinolytics).

- hormones (oestrogen, progestogen, oral contraception, GnRH analogues).

Mirena® IUS – hormonal method consisting of a frame with a hormonal sleeve, providing local delivery of a progestogen (levonorgestrel). This requires a procedure for insertion and is normally done in a clinic setting. For most women insertion is a simple procedure, not requiring any form of anaesthetic although local anaesthetic can make a difference. A very small number of women require a brief general anaesthetic.

SURGERY

Hysterectomy

If the uterus is removed, then this is a hysterectomy which can be done abdominally through a "bikini" incision or vaginally leaving no visible scar. There must be a scar of course and this is at the top of the vagina. No external scarring does not mean that a major operation has not taken place and recovery, particularly with regard to lifting, can take up to 12 weeks. Hysterectomy can also be done laparoscopically using a minimally invasive technique also known as keyhole surgery. There are then usually three small scars on the abdomen plus the scar at the top of the vagina.

One decision has to be made prior to the operation and this is whether the ovaries should be removed or left behind (conserved). If they are left in, the hormone cycle continues and so disorders which depend on that cycle will not be treated. These include premenstrual syndrome (PMS) and endometriosis. If the ovaries are removed then this will create a surgical menopause, resulting in the symptoms outlined in Chapter 11. Of course the consequences of the menopause then begin at a younger age and must be considered – particularly osteoporosis. Menopausal problems can be prevented by appropriate hormone replacement and a woman having her ovaries removed at 35, for example, will need replacement therapy at least until the average age of menopause, 51–52. Under these circumstances, HRT is NOT associated with the risks that are said to occur when treatment is initiated later in life, after the natural menopause. It is much easier to avoid hysterectomy in this day and age either by medical treatment or endometrial ablation.

Endometrial Ablation

As a young junior doctor in 1974, I (PMSOB) had just used a cryocautery – freezing – probe to treat a small benign lesion (an erosion) on the cervix – this works by freezing, to remove the superficial abnormal tissue and then normal tissue grows over. I suggested to the more senior doctor (a lecturer) that we should devise a probe to similarly destroy the tissue of the endometrial lining and set up a study to see if we could stop or reduce periods and avoid the need for hysterectomy. He was not impressed by this idea, suggesting it would not work and would not catch on. He was wrong – there are now countless methods for ablating the endometrium, including cryocauterisation.

I should point out that the amazing, inspirational archetypal Australian gynaecologist had previously just taught me to do the cryocautery to the cervix and instructed me to say to the patients just before the freezing probe was applied to the cervix that the procedure "Does not hurt at all, it is just a bit like making love to an Eskimo" – just how much political incorrectness can you get into eight words?

The other endometrial ablation methods include virtually every modern day energy source – microwave ablation, radiofrequency, electrical current, electrical cautery, hot water and so on. If there are many different ways of treating something that usually is because none is perfect, either from the point of view of efficacy or the risk of unwanted effects or complications. The important things from a hormonal point of view are as follows. Firstly, it may not work and so other medical treatment or surgery may ultimately be required. Following ablation, not every bit of endometrial tissue is destroyed and so when hormone replacement therapy is required it is still necessary to give both oestrogen and a progestogen to avoid the risk of cancer of the endometrium. Finally, there only needs to a small amount of the endometrium for a pregnancy to occur and PMSOB reported such a case in the *Journal of Obstetrics and Gynaecology* in 1994. So that means that contraception or sterilisation is still necessary.

MEDICAL TREATMENT OF HEAVY PERIODS
In the information already provided, we hope we suggested that surgery may be avoidable if medical treatment, which is preferable, is successful. All women should access some form of treatment, so if it seems like we are repeating ourselves, we are because this is so important!

Medical treatments include:

Use of drugs which affect the prostaglandins, controlling the bleeding from blood vessels (non-steroidals).

Drugs which affect coagulation mechanisms (antifibrinolytics).

Use of hormones (oestrogen, progestogen, oral contraception, GnRH analogues).

Let's discuss each in reasonable detail. You will realise by now that many drugs used for one disorder are also used for others, either relying on the same or a different mechanism.

Non-steroidals
These are the non-steroidal anti-inflammatory group of drugs (NSAIDS). Sounds complicated, but basically they stop the synthesis of the tiny local chemical messengers,

the prostaglandins. Some of these drugs are everyday anti-inflammatory and pain relieving drugs, which you will have used to nurse a rugby injury or a hangover (perhaps both at the same time!), Aspirin, Brufen, Nurofen and so forth. For many years, women have been prescribed another one called Mefenamic acid or Ponstan® for painful periods. This is more powerful and is very effective, at least for painful periods. Contract your biceps now very tightly and hold it there for a long time. The blood supply is reduced and this with the prolonged muscle contraction, combine to give pain – a period pain works similarly to this. Prostaglandins are released in relation to the pain of inflammation caused by contraction of the muscle of the uterus, with a reduction of blood supply. It was also found that the use of mefenamic acid reduced menstrual blood loss, probably by closing the blood vessels which become exposed after shedding of the endometrial lining. Again this is due to blocking prostaglandin release but we do not think we should try and explain it as we do not understand it sufficiently ourselves – suffice to say mefenamic acid blocks the prostaglandins which normally keep the blood vessels open - they close and the bleeding is reduced.

As many women have both painful and heavy periods, this drug can be very useful and it only needs to be taken during the period.

Drugs controlling Coagulation

There are only a few things more complicated than blood clotting factors and mechanisms. In relation to heavy menstrual bleeding, we need to understand that tranexamic acid prevents the chemical that prevents blood clotting from happening i.e. it lets the blood clotting happen effectively, thus reducing bleeding. It is reasonably effective in some women and has few side effects (it is sold over the counter in Scandinavia and we would not be surprised if one day that will be the case in the UK as well). This drug also only needs to be taken during the heavy days of menstrual bleeding, ideally in sufficient quantities to ensure that it has the desired effect. Patients are normally recommended to take two tablets four times a day for the first four days of bleeding or longer if the bleeding is still heavy.

Hormone Treatment

Hormones can be used to stop the menstrual cycle, regulate it, or reduce the volume, duration and frequency of bleeding. You have already heard about some of these hormones and as stated previously the same hormones can be used for different purposes. Taking the oral contraceptive ("pill") for instance, reduces bleeding and pain as a welcome non-contraceptive benefit. It first came to market in the 1960s as a method of contraception. Quite high doses of hormones were used and side effects were more common than they are with the low dose pills we use nowadays. When it was first designed, the idea was to give relatively high doses of both oestrogen and progestogen in order to override the central (pituitary gland) control of the cycle. Remember in Chapter 2 we described the two hormones FSH and LH as being necessary to control the cycle – this resulted in the production of oestrogen, then the development and release of the egg followed by the production of progesterone for the second half of the cycle. If we administer oestrogen and progesterone-like hormones, known as progestogens, to women in sufficient doses, this in effect sends a signal to the pituitary gland that there is sufficient hormone and there is no need to produce any more LH or FSH. But LH is necessary to stimulate ovulation – without it, no ovulation cycle, no egg and no pregnancy.

If the contraceptive pill was to be given continuously there would not be an endometrial cycle either – so no endometrial build up – no bleeding. In the early development of the pill it was felt that a monthly bleed would be more acceptable to women (women say that "men would think that wouldn't they?!") and it was probably better to have a break to reassure women of the contraceptive effect, when their "period" came. So it was designed with three weeks of combined hormone with a one week break. It was soon found that giving the pill reduced periods significantly and it has been used extensively for this purpose ever since. In 1974 a study by the Royal College of General Practitioners suggested that women over 35 were at increased risk of heart attacks and strokes and this led to the pill being withheld for these women. However, the results of the study actually only showed this to be a problem in smokers, but the anxiety has persisted amongst GPs who are often still reluctant to prescribe this very effective method of contraception to women over 35, the group most likely to have heavy periods.

Actually giving the pill without a break is even more effective and can treat many of the other conditions in addition to heavy periods. These include conditions such as painful periods, endometriosis, PMS (possibly), and pelvic pain. It is most important that women are reassured that menstrual blood is not building up and will not "explode" at some inappropriate moment, for example in the middle of the supermarket. In women taking the pill continuously without a break there is no build-up of the endometrial lining and less, if anything, to shed.

So, very many women have the potential to benefit from taking the pill. Only those with a personal history of migraine with aura, a family history of deep vein thrombosis (blood clots in the leg or the lung) in first degree relatives below the age of 45, smokers over 35 and women taking medication which stimulates liver metabolism reducing the effectiveness of the pill need special consideration. The pill should not be prescribed to women without first checking blood pressure or body mass index, both of which should be normal.

Progestogen Treatment
GPs have prescribed these drugs (norethisterone and medroxyprogesterone acetate) for many years. They have followed the manufacturers guidance to the letter and given the treatment for two weeks out of four. Research shows that these

drugs (specifically norethisterone) work best if given in higher doses (15 mg rather than 10mg) and for three weeks (not two) out of four or even continuously in the short term until a long term solution can be found. It is also important to note that very often the drugs can induce for the first time symptoms of PMS. This is not well known, but understanding potential side effects can help women persevere in order to benefit from long term effective treatment. Progestogens given as we have suggested are often effective and are worth a try.

Danazol

This drug was used for endometriosis, but can also be effective for cyclical breast pain, PMS and heavy periods. It is taken every day. We said earlier that the differences between the various male and female hormones is not great – a sort of spectrum between maleness and femaleness. Danazol is a bit more towards the male side and so can have side effects of masculinisation – this is particularly important because most drugs given for heavy periods will be given for a long period of time. The sort of problems seen are acne and weight gain and if high doses are given for a long time, hirsutism (male distribution and facial hair) can occur as well as deepening of the voice. If the periods improve with low doses, then it may still be a useful drug.

It is not prescribed often these days because of the fear of these side effects which is a shame because it can be very effective, especially if your woman wants to turn into a man!

GnRH analogues

Remember there are several of these drugs and they can be taken nasally or by injection. Remember also that they cause a temporary menopause-like state and so they are rarely used for heavy periods for a long time. They nearly always stop periods though and there are situations where they can be used for around six months.

GnRH analogues can be helpful in women waiting for surgery, especially in women with anaemia (caused by excessive bleeding) as this will give the body a chance to recover before surgery, possibly avoiding the need for a blood transfusion.

We have talked about hysterectomy and endometrial ablation. Let's briefly explain what is meant by pelvic ultrasound, hysteroscopy, and endometrial biopsy because many women being investigated for hormonal problems could need one or more of these procedures at some point.

Pelvic ultrasound scan

Ultrasound is a very valuable investigation, particularly using a transvaginal approach. All of the female pelvic organs can be visualised in this way, unless there are limiting factors, the most common of which is obesity.

Ultrasound is particularly useful for diagnosing fibroids, endometrial polyps, endometrial cancer and other uterine abnormalities, polycystic ovaries, ovarian cysts and ovarian cancer. Unfortunately, it is not very useful for diagnosing endometriosis unless there are associated chocolate cysts (not real chocolate but altered blood cysts - endometriomas). Transvaginal ultrasound is not painful and women should not worry about having this investigation. Ideally the result should be discussed with the patient at the time of the procedure to reduce anxiety.

Hysteroscopy

This is a simple investigation that is most often done in an outpatient setting with the patient awake. The uterine cavity is inspected with a hysteroscope, which is a thin camera that can be passed through the narrow opening in the cervix, allowing inspection of the inside of the uterus. It can be combined with removal of polyps, a biopsy and insertion of Mirena® if the patient wishes.

Complications are not common, but include bleeding, infection and more rarely perforation (a hole through the uterus) requiring admission, antibiotics and very, very rarely a laparoscopy if bleeding into the pelvis is suspected.

Occasionally hysteroscopy will be performed under general anaesthetic, usually if the patient is unable to tolerate it awake. The objectives include determining the cause of bleeding and the exclusion of cancer of the endometrium in, for example, women with postmenopausal or perimenopausal bleeding.

Endometrial biopsy
This is a relatively simple technique, requiring skills and equipment similar to inserting an intrauterine contraceptive device. It is not a comfortable procedure but is quick and enables tissue to be collected from inside the womb and cancer to be excluded.

Professor Shaughn O'Brien & Dr Paula Briggs

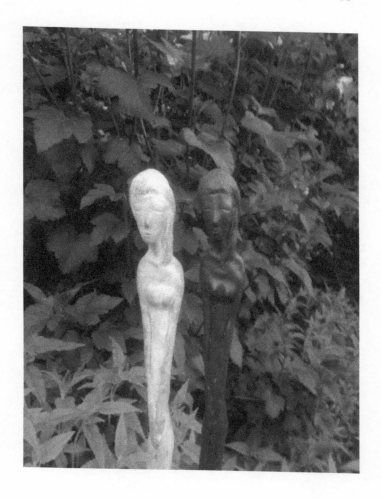

Two Sides of a Young Woman 2014

CHAPTER 7

Premenstrual Syndrome

In this chapter:

What is it?

Who gets it?

What are the symptoms?

What are the effects of PMS?

What are the terms used?

How is it measured?

The PreMentricS app for diagnosis

What is the cause?

How is it treated?
    Non-drug
    Non-hormonal drugs
    Hormones

Can surgery be justified?

Premenstrual syndrome. You will have noticed by now that these chapters are pretty short. That's because they are written for men, who tend usually to have spatial ability and not verbal – that is they prefer pictures! We have established that negative symptoms in relation to hormones, before the menopause, are almost certainly innate, occurring naturally. These symptoms might have been beneficial in the history of our species (Chapter 14), but persist now their purpose has long gone. This is not a particular problem when the symptoms are mild, but when severe they can be incredibly destructive to the woman's (and man's!) life, normal functioning and work. Conditions such as PMS can significantly impact on the lives of those around the affected women such as colleagues, children and husbands. It can ruin marriages. Only 5% of women (in their reproductive years) have absolutely no premenstrual symptoms. Another 5% fall at the other extreme, with very significant symptoms.

PMS is referred to as PMDD (premenstrual dysphoric disorder) by American Psychiatrists and relates to the extreme psychological part of the symptom spectrum. This may eventually become the term used in the UK and Europe, but we suspect not. Many women now use the term to persuade their GPs that they have a *real* condition, when they have previously been ignored and told it is 'a woman's lot'.

Of course, there is a wide spectrum or range of premenstrual symptoms, between badly affected women and those with no symptoms. Where you draw the line between normal and abnormal may be difficult and arbitrary.

What are the symptoms? Well, Jekyll and Hyde has been mentioned. One of us (PMSOB) once gave a lecture to a group of doctors in Riyadh, Saudi Arabia – unfortunately, he spent most of the lecture trying to explain who Jekyll and Hyde were and on reaching the end of the lecture there were loud comments that PMS did not exist and was not a problem – well that was what the male trainees said –the female trainees all came up to him and quietly contradicted this. Some symptoms of PMS are common to most women. Others are unique to an individual woman but, by definition, they occur specifically in the premenstrual phase of her cycle.

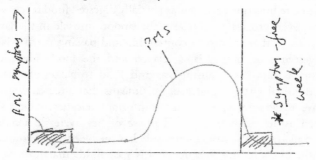

Figure 11

The symptoms of PMS/PMDD typically follow the pattern of progesterone production (see Figure 6).

Everyone knows the symptoms of PMS, or do they? They can be physical or psychological. Common physical symptoms include breast swelling, tenderness and bloating. These can be extreme, distressing and intolerable. A patient once requested removal of her breasts for no other reason than cyclical breast pain. Abdominal bloating can also be a very distressing symptom. Some women need to wear clothing two sizes bigger premenstrually. The cause of bloating is difficult to define. It was originally thought to be due to water retention, but this is now thought to be unlikely, so the use of diuretics would be nonsense, in all but a few women. Although some women do put on weight, many women become bloated without doing so. It is impossible to retain water without gaining weight and so in the majority of women who become distressingly distended without an increase in weight, my suggestion is that this is mainly due to distension of the bowel with gas.

We saw in Chapter 2 that the hormone progesterone (the one produced after ovulation in the second half of the cycle) causes relaxation of certain types of muscle (smooth muscle) which is found in many different organs. Remember that smooth muscle contracts without our control, not like the biceps, or quads, but in response to physical or chemical change – for instance full bladder, full bowel and so forth. Normally the large intestine contracts as partially digested food reaches it. However, progesterone relaxes the smooth muscle in the large bowel, so that instead of contracting and passing the partially digested food along, it is relaxed and the food substances remain stationary, causing gas and fluid to accumulate and abdominal girth to increase. This means that affected women have to choose bigger, more comfortable clothes, which she then associates with the bad phase of her cycle. When her period arrives the woman not only has the bleeding to contend with, but also the loss of all this gas, fluid, diarrhoea with associated bowel cramps and period pains. She may say "Next time I am coming back as a man" – however she would have to put up with the major disadvantage of having to read this book! By the end of her period, it is as if a cloud has lifted – the bleeding has stopped, the pain has gone, her breasts return to their normal size and she feels comfortable again. With the bloating completely gone she can get into jeans, and feel like an attractive member of the female species again.

That is just the physical symptoms. Some women only get the physical ones – others only get the mood and psychological ones – many really unlucky women get both!

The psychological symptoms can be the most distressing. First imagine you are a woman! Now imagine that for up to two weeks of every month, hormones cause changes to your body over which you have no immediate control. For no obvious reason your world seems to take on a very negative outlook – you are depressed, crying, feel unloved, you do not like your husband or children, all of whom are getting on your nerves as never before. You might want to hit your husband and may even do so, after which you will feel regret and remorse. You are out of control, you want to hit your children and if you do, you will feel absolutely dreadful about it. You feel ugly, spotty, fat and bloated, with a puffy face. You are tired, weak, clumsy, forgetful and useless. Your family and people in work do not understand and not surprisingly they begin to find you and your actions intolerable. No one feels sorry for you either, of course!

This was exactly how you felt last month, but once you feel better you do not remember just how distressed you were. It's as though it never happened, until next time. Then it starts again, its hell on earth for everyone.

Now, return to being a man again – why should you have to make adjustments for her irrational behaviour?

A good way to measure symptoms and see the relationship to the cycle is to use the PreMenstricS app.

Remember that if a woman was reading this book – and they have been warned not to – she may wonder how one man and one woman can have so much insight into how other women think – many women have precisely the pattern and character of symptoms we have described (some, if not all). Other women will state that we are talking a lot of nonsense because that is not what they experience. However, the majority of women with true PMS will empathise with this view and we have had the professional life long opportunity of the second hand experience of many thousands of women.

Some women will not have PMS at all. One woman (aged 71) who spoke to me (PMSOB) on a radio phone-in programme said that in her day she just had to put up with it, and the women of today simply have not learned to cope. She clearly did not have PMS, rather premenstrual symptoms. She was very unaccepting of women with severe symptoms. Some women have symptoms, which don't disappear after their period. Again these women do not have PMS, rather a continuous low mood/depression or another psychological disorder. As their condition has nothing to do with hormones at all, these women will be very dissatisfied with GPs, PMS experts, their husbands and life in general. The last group of unsympathetic women, are those with no symptoms at all (5% of the female population). No one worries too much if these women deny the existence of PMS, as long as it's not your partner's GP! Then you and your woman are in trouble. If certain women were to read this book, then they might be very critical that I am trying to "medicalise women's menstrual cycles" or trying to use PMS pejoratively in the interest of men! Firstly, they should not be reading this book, and secondly they should be talking to affected women and not extrapolating their own narrow experiences to other women.

Professor Shaughn O'Brien & Dr Paula Briggs

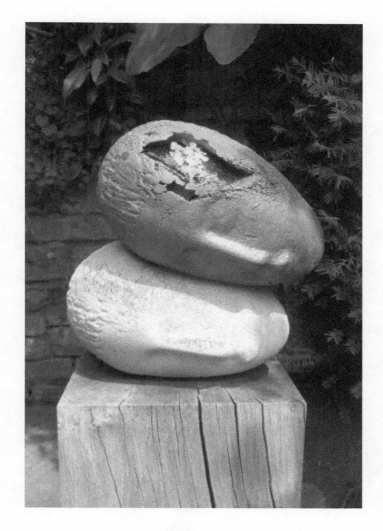

Resolution 2019

CHAPTER 8

Treatment of PMS

Effective treatments for PMS do exist although currently there are no licensed treatments available in the UK. There are many unlicensed approaches – some very effective.

Firstly, it is important to review the likely cause of the problem.

In simple terms the problem is caused by *normal* hormone levels in women in whom their brains are *excessively sensitive* to the hormone progesterone, produced by the ovary after ovulation. So the treatment options include either:

    a. Reducing the sensitivity of brain receptors to the progesterone

    b. Stopping ovulation which will prevent the production of progesterone

a. Reducing Brain Receptor Sensitivity

There are many types of receptors in the brain and there are many drugs that can influence them. Serotonin receptors are linked to depression and PMS. The use of drugs which increase of serotonin and decrease sensitivity to progesterone are effective. You will have heard of Prozac/fluoxetine – and maybe other similar drugs including citalopram, sertraline and more. GPs freely prescribe these but for some reason avoid prescribing hormones. They can be very effective and are licensed in the US to treat PMDD. However, they can reduce sex-drive and orgasm. Side effects can be minimised by use just in the second half of the cycle. They certainly don't work for all affected women but can result in a successful outcome in others. When a patient gets to see a gynaecologist it is usually only after these drugs have failed.

b. Stopping Ovulation

This can be achieved in several ways. Generally speaking, hormones are used to block or change the natural cycle and eliminate ovulation. The main difficulty is that if the hormone cycle is stopped completely, that will create an early artificial menopause with all the connected symptoms and risks (hot flushes, increased risk of heart disease and osteoporosis). The hormone oestrogen can be used to stop ovulation, but if it is used on its own, that risks causing cancer of the lining of the uterus. This can be prevented by giving a progestogen, but we already know that this class of hormone is the cause of the PMS in the first place.

Most people know that the combined pill works by stopping ovulation. So, seemingly, it should treat PMS, because ovulation is suppressed. However, because it contains progestogen, PMS symptoms are frequently reintroduced. There may be one pill (Yaz® in the US/Eloine® in the UK) which can stop ovulation without bringing back PMS symptoms in some women. Some progestogen-only pills stop ovulation, but they have a high risk of causing PMS-like symptoms continuously.

Stopping ovulation can be achieved by using oestrogen (transdermally) as patches and gels or subcutaneously as implants.

This is very effective for treating PMS symptoms, but as we have already said oestrogen alone can cause cancer of the lining of the uterus. This can be prevented by progestogen, but with the likely return of PMS. A clever way around this is as follows.

Oestrogen is given transdermally in sufficient doses to stop ovulation (more than HRT; less than the pill). Progestogen is then given to protect the uterine lining from cancer. An oral progestogen should be tried first and this can be successful for some patients. However, if it does bring back the PMS, then the progestogen can be inserted into the uterus (Mirena®), with maximal effect due to proximity to the endometrium, but minimal side effects due to low levels absorbed into the blood stream. Very many of our patients have been successfully treated in this way for many years.

Many women over 40 who may be approaching the menopause, have worsening PMS, have heavy periods and are beginning to have hot flushes. They may also be worried about their contraception. The combination of oestrogen and Mirena® has the ability to solve all of these problems in one package!

Warning: just occasionally some patients absorb the hormone delivered directly to the endometrial cavity into the bloodstream and it influences the receptors in the brain and gives continuous PMS-like symptoms. Fortunately, Mirena® can easily be removed in these circumstances. The second important part of this warning is that very few GPs, psychiatrists and even gynaecologists are aware of this possibility! The third part of the warning is that you shouldn't remove the Mirena® too quickly, if at all possible, as this side effect may be transient.

GnRH ANALOGUES

If you stop the hormone cycle completely, all PMS symptoms will disappear.

Drugs such as Prostap® and Zoladex® are injected usually as a 12-week depot (long acting pellet or depot placed in the fatty tissue under the skin).

This creates a chemically-induced temporary menopause. Menopausal symptoms will usually develop and in the long term, there is the risk of bone thinning or osteoporosis. These symptoms can be prevented by giving add-back HRT, but then of course we return to all of the issues associated with the need for a progestogen to protect the lining of the womb, highlighted in the previous paragraph.

Several years ago the first clinic was set up for both PMS and the menopause.

The first half of the clinic was spent stopping the hormone cycle to treat PMS symptoms, but causing menopause symptoms and the second half of the clinic was spent giving hormones to treat the menopause, which caused PMS!

You have probably worked out by now that the key obstacle to the management of PMS is how to protect the lining of the uterus – the endometrium.

- When hormone cycles are normal, the lining of the uterus builds up and sheds every month, with no risk of cancer.

- If all the hormones are all suppressed, the lining of the uterus thins with no risk of cancer, but the rest of the body suffers as a result of hormone deficiency side effects, which are identical to symptoms of menopause.

- If we give just oestrogen, the hormone cycle is suppressed, there are no PMS symptoms, but without a progestogen there is a higher risk of cancer of the womb.

- If we add a progestogen, we protect the endometrium from cancer, but the PMS symptoms are likely to return.

- If there was no endometrium, we could give oestrogen to suppress the cycle and eliminate PMS, without any need to give progestogen.

The only way to remove the endometrium is by hysterectomy. Endometrial ablation, as we have said in an earlier chapter, may not remove it all, so that (a) contraception is still required and (b) as before, progestogen is still required to protect the endometrium.

If your wife/partner is considering surgery and wishes you to help her talk through the decision, then I think you could let her see this part of the book with the following list of facts that need to be thought through.

- Removing the uterus will prevent all chances of having (further) children.

- It is a major operation with known complications.

- However, it can be done these days by keyhole surgery.

- If only the uterus is removed, the ovaries will remain as will the hormone cycles, which will mean continued PMS. But this could be suppressed with oestrogen treatment, without progestogen. From our clinical experience this is not usually a good plan.

- Removing just the ovaries is nearly always verging on daft, because oestrogen will be required to prevent osteoporosis and the endometrium will require progestogen, the source of the problem in the first place! Beware, some laparoscopic surgeons like to do this easier operation!

The only natural cure for PMS is to reach the menopause! More later!

The only permanent medical cure is surgery and this in our long experience should be removal of the uterus including the cervix, both tubes and ovaries, undertaken ideally by keyhole surgery; Surgery will be followed by oestrogen replacement with no need for progestogen – i.e. laparoscopic total hysterectomy and bilateral salpingo-oophorectomy with unopposed oestrogen replacement therapy. It would be wise to have a "test drive" before committing as follows:

- Create a temporary medical menopause using a GnRH analogue.

- Give oestrogen-only add-back (safe without progestogen short term).

- Symptoms related to the hormone cycle will disappear and there will be no menopausal symptoms. This regimen will *not* remove the symptoms of any underlying mood disorder unrelated to PMS – what goes and stays with the "test drive" will go and stay after the surgery.

NON-DRUG
There are many non-drug treatments and probably the best of these is CBT or Cognitive Behavioural Therapy. If Prozac-like drugs and hormones are to be avoided, then probably this should be the first step. As this book is intended to be about hormones and not alternative therapy, we will say no more but further information can be gathered from the National Association for PMS or the Royal College of Obstetricians and Gynaecologists Guideline.

These are easily accessed
Google: 'RCOG 48' Or www.pms.org

THE FUTURE
The future for PMS/PMDD treatment will be improved by the increasing acceptance and awareness of the condition by the media, general public and the medical profession which is happening now. Also, the development of new treatment strategies will be important.

HOT OFF THE PRESS
1. Since writing this book, the World Health Organisation (WHO) has recognized officially the term PMDD as being the extreme psychological end of Premenstrual Syndrome spectrum.

2. Research on the drug Sepranolone, the new drug especially developed for specifically PMDD, has probably not been proven, as hoped, to be more effective than placebo for the management of the disorder.

Professor Shaughn O'Brien & Dr Paula Briggs

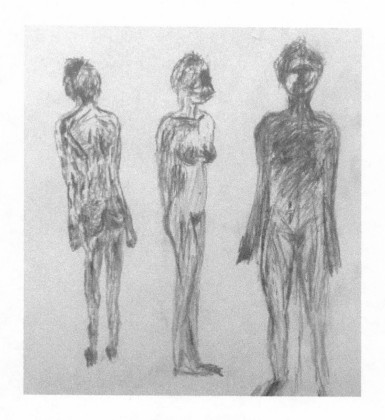

Preliminary sketches 2019

HerHormones

CHAPTER 9

Polycystic ovaries and polycystic ovary syndrome – what's the difference?

Around 20% of women have a polycystic pattern on ultrasound examination of their ovaries. This is not a medical finding, rather a normal finding – just your woman's ovaries. However, approximately half of women with this type of ovary will have the syndrome, as defined by a consensus on diagnostic standards, known as the Rotterdam Criteria.

A polycystic ovary (PCO), when viewed by the naked eye, is seen to have an increased number of small follicles – fluid filled "pseudocysts". These are not "cysts" and certainly do not require an operation. They are not a cause of pelvic pain. Each small follicle contains an egg, capable of developing into a pregnancy. The terminology is confusing for women (and men), especially for those with just polycystic ovaries without the syndrome, who then perceive their normal ovaries to be diseased.

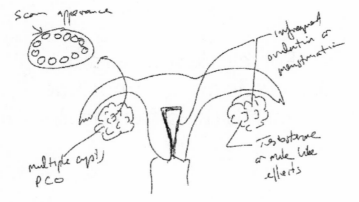

Figure 12

In women with polycystic ovaries, the ovaries enlarge and have many small cysts. The hormonal pattern becomes disrupted so that ovulation may not occur (infertility and infrequent heavy periods), and there may be an increase in testosterone causing problems such as hirsutism (exaggerated hairiness, acne and occasionally male pattern baldness).

The characteristic polycystic ovaries can be seen on ultrasound scan. Just polycystic ovaries is not problem.

With infrequent periods/ovulation or with testosterone effects it is called Polycystic Ovary Syndrome (PCOS).

The diagnostic criteria agreed by consensus in 2003, concluded that a diagnosis of polycystic ovary syndrome (PCOS) could be made where features include any two of the following three characteristics:

1. **Infrequent menstrual bleeding** (infrequent periods) – this is because women with this type of ovary do not produce an egg every month and some may do so very infrequently. When bleeding does it occur, it can be very heavy. This is because the lining of the uterus becomes too thick. This is not good for women and if left untreated can increase the risk of cancer. The other problem for women releasing an egg infrequently is that there may be difficulty becoming pregnant. It is important to point out however, that women who do not want a pregnancy, should never rely on

infrequent egg release as a means of contraception. Nature has a wicked sense of humour!

2. **Polycystic ovaries on ultrasound** – these are larger than "normal" ovaries with peripheral cysts, which have the appearance of a string of black pearls. The volume if measured is greater than 10 cubic centimetres.

3. **Clinical findings (acne or hairiness (hirsutism)** and/ or blood tests showing **high levels** of what are normally thought of as **male hormones** (androgens).

Although women meeting these criteria are most likely to have PCOS, there are a number of other conditions relating to endocrine glands, which should be ruled out and therefore management by a reproductive health specialist is recommended. PCOS although common, is a complex endocrine (hormonal) condition with significant health risks. Many affected women are also overweight and at risk of becoming type 2 diabetics. Although commonly associated with PCOS, neither is a requirement for diagnosis.

So, an ultrasound scan is not actually necessary to make a diagnosis of PCOS. However, it is good for assessing the lining of the womb, which as we said, can become too thick [It is strange that the criteria place a woman with and without polycystic ovaries on scan in seemingly odd categories. Theoretically, she can have polycystic ovaries (only) and not have PCOS but can actually have PCOS (two of the other criteria) but with normal ovaries].

We are now going to try to explain what goes wrong in women with PCOS and then think about potential management options for this condition.

The management plan for any affected woman should be based on her presenting problem e.g. infrequent but heavy bleeding, clinical symptoms associated with excess androgens ('male' hormones) – acne and/or hairiness (hirsutism) or difficulty getting pregnant. Women who don't want to become pregnant should use reliable contraception and there are methods, which can be safely used, including those with added benefits, e.g. Mirena® which will protect the lining of the womb from cancer and reduce bleeding and others where the hormone antagonises the 'male' hormone (e.g. pills containing cyproterone acetate like Dianette®). For some women with PCOS the combined pill might not be advisable. For example, in women who are significantly overweight or who have an increase in the risk of blood clots.

UNDERSTANDING WHAT GOES WRONG IN PCOS (IN OUTLINE AND THEN HOW TO DEAL WITH THE PROBLEM

This will depend on an individual risk assessment including a detailed history, examination and possibly some investigations, which will include an ultrasound scan and blood tests.

All sex steroid hormones are derived from cholesterol, which you will likely recognise as a fat. Women with PCOS have a hormone imbalance and they make more "male" hormones, which coincidentally perpetuates the polycystic appearance of the ovary. Yes, ovaries can change their appearance and behaviour, just like women! Now for sex hormone binding globulin (SHBG), which binds male hormones, "mops them up" like a sponge, reducing the level of freely available "male" hormone and thus its actions – the root cause of the problem in women with PCOS. SHBG levels are inversely proportional to body weight and as women with PCOS are often overweight, they frequently have a lower level of SHBG (a smaller sponge), with an increase in the amount of free or "active" circulating androgens. This further exacerbates the clinical features of PCOS. Insulin resistance is common in women with PCOS, particularly those who are overweight, and can be a precursor to impaired glucose tolerance (this means that there is a risk of developing diabetes). Weight reduction will reduce the likelihood of insulin resistance occurring and also increase the level of SHBG "sponge", reducing free androgens. In addition, as insulin is an anabolic steroid (vaguely similar to those used by body building sportsmen) it is associated with weight gain, consequently reducing the size of the sponge, increasing free androgen levels, perpetuating the problem. A higher level of insulin also has a direct effect on hepatic (liver) synthesis of SHBG, reducing the size of the "sponge", further increasing the unbound circulating androgens – i.e. it is acting as a "multiplier".

In summary, the drivers for increased ovarian androgen production in women with PCOS include a hormone imbalance, obesity and higher insulin levels.

For overweight women with PCOS, weight loss is the most important element of management. Once the body mass index is below 30, fertility improves and contraception becomes much more important.

BELOW ARE SOME CHOICES TO HELP MANAGE THE SYMPTOMS OF PCOS

Generally, this will depend on what the problem is:

BUT

All women with PCOS should be advised regarding diet and exercise

Infrequent and/or heavy menstrual bleeding and symptoms of excess androgens:

a. Mirena ® for endometrial protection and contraception
    Cyproterone acetate can be prescribed separately
    in a dose of 25 mg daily to block the male
    hormone receptor.

or

b. Combined hormonal contraception – pill, patch or vaginal ring dependent upon individual preference and a risk assessment to exclude contraindications.
   - Women with acne or excess hair can benefit from the use of pills which contain a progestogen which blocks the male hormone, e.g. cyproterone acetate in Dianette® or drospirenone in Eloine® and Yasmin®

c. For those women who decline a Mirena® and who have contraindications to oestrogen e.g. a BMI > 40, a mini pill e.g. Cerazette® or equivalent can be provided both for protection of the lining of the womb and contraception. A contraceptive implant is another possible choice but neither of these have a male hormone blocking effect.

Fertility: A common misconception is that women with PCOS will not be able to conceive. This is not the case and contraception is particularly important both for its non-contraceptive benefits as outlined above and to control fertility/plan pregnancies appropriately.

For women struggling to get pregnant, there are a variety of assisted conception options.

These include several methods of ovulation stimulation and they need to be undertaken with fairly strict clinical surveillance to avoid hyperstimulation of the ovaries and multiple pregnancies.

For further advice, the PCOS patient website can be useful: www.verity-pcos.org.uk

Professor Shaughn O'Brien & Dr Paula Briggs

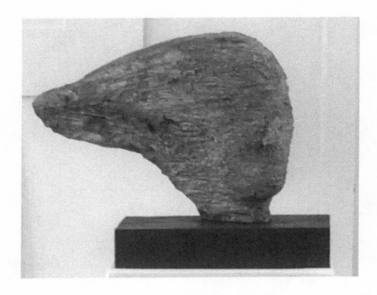

Challenge in a Different Guise 2019

HerHormones

CHAPTER 10

Endometriosis

Endometriosis is quite common and can occur at any phase throughout reproductive life. It can result in heavy painful periods (dysmenorrhoea), painful penetrative sex (deep dyspareunia), poor quality of life and possible subfertility.

WHAT IS ENDOMETRIOSIS?

We have seen that the lining of the uterus/endometrium builds up through the course of the menstrual cycle and then breaks down and the tissue is shed - a period. Endometriosis is similar to this but the tissue is in the wrong location and so the shedding occurs in the wrong site causing pain, inflammation and the development of, potentially, very damaging scar tissue. There are common places where the tissue develops, including the ovaries (where it may cause ovarian [chocolate] cysts), the fallopian tubes (where it may cause fertility problems), anywhere in the lining tissue of the pelvis (peritoneum), down between the uterus and the rectum (the pouch of Douglas), the bladder, and the cervix.

It can actually be within the muscle of the uterus where it is called *adenomyosis*.

More rarely is can occur in the umbilicus causing monthly bleeding from the navel; in the nose causing monthly nose bleeds; in the lungs causing monthly coughing of blood and lung collapse. Occasionally tissue can get deposited in the scar of a caesarean section which will give monthly scar pain when the periods return. Medical students find these rare sites very interesting, but it is far more important to concentrate on the common ones.

Essentially endometriosis is a common condition which rarely has anything to do with cancer. Blood tests do not help with the diagnosis; scans are pretty unhelpful; x-ray is not usually indicated; MRI is particularly valuable in certain circumstances, for example where there is endometriosis is located way down between the rectum and vagina, when this has been missed at laparoscopy. Laparoscopy is a keyhole or minimally invasive investigation which is in most cases the gold standard diagnostic technique. These days it is usually combined with the possibility of progressing immediately to surgical treatment.

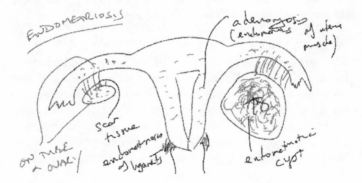

Figure 13

Endometriosis is very common. Tissue like that of the endometrium develops or becomes located in other sites such as the ovary, tube, cervix, uterine wall, lining of the pelvis and occasionally beyond the pelvis (nose, lung, umbilicus). It is not surprising that all this can be associated with painful periods, painful sex and infertility.

THE SYMPTOMS OF ENDOMETRIOSIS

There are what we would describe as usual endometriosis symptoms:

Subfertility can occur due to damage to the pelvis and fallopian tubes, preventing the sperm from reaching the egg.

Women may experience extreme pain during sexual intercourse, with deep penetration leading to avoidance. There are of course ways of experiencing sexual activity without deep penetration and men need to be sensitive to this as it can cause a lot of marital stress.

Severe period pain tends to start as the period approaches and continues throughout the bleed but sometimes not for the duration of bleeding.

Early diagnosis and treatment can reduce the risk of pain, suffering and irreversible damage to the pelvis and Fallopian tubes.

TREATMENT

As with many of the conditions described in this book stopping the ovarian hormone cycle can result in eradication of the symptoms. If we can stop bleeding from the uterus (no period), then it is very unlikely that the site of the wrongly located endometriotic tissue will bleed.

If the pill is taken without the usual break, then the withdrawal bleed does not occur. Progestogens (progesterone-like synthetic hormones) prevent the endometrium and the endometriosis from proliferating. Danazol was frequently used in the past, but rarely if ever now due to the side effects of masculinisation – remember how the "chicken-wire" structure of the sex steroid hormones requires only subtle substitutions for marked differences in effect and the repercussions of treatment with danazol lie somewhere between those associated with progesterone and testosterone.

The GnRH drugs are usually injected depots and stop the ovarian cycle right at the central point i.e. by suppressing the pituitary gland (control box). Of course, this will cause all the side effects of the menopause and so it should not normally be a long term solution.

Surgical treatment can be conservative i.e. only removing the endometriotic tissue and scar tissue or is can be definitive by removing the uterus, tubes and ovaries in addition to all deposits of endometriosis and scar tissue in the pelvis. Conservative treatment can be followed by recurrence.

Extensive endometriosis may rarely require surgery to bowel, bladder or wherever else is involved and definitive surgery is usually a last resort. Also of course coming into play is reproductive history, desire for (further) children and how effective the prior medical approaches have been.

Professor Shaughn O'Brien & Dr Paula Briggs

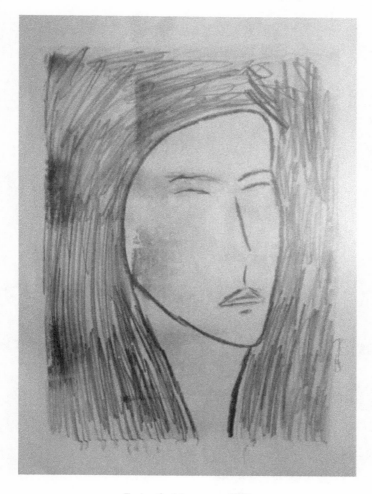

Facing the Menopause 2019

HerHormones

CHAPTER 11

The Menopause Defined

Introduction

What is the menopause?

Who "gets it"?

What are the symptoms?

Do all women get symptoms?

What are the unknowns?

And most importantly, how does the menopause affect a woman's partner?

What men can do to help

What help is available for men?

If there is one area of women's health that causes more anguish than any other, it is the menopause. This is not simply the "condition" itself, but the media's response to research. Remember the media do not produce articles just because of public interest. Articles in newspapers are there for the journalist's and the newspapers interest – essentially to fill the spaces between the ads and to sell more newspapers! So there is no purpose in a headline that says "HRT is Safe". A headline saying HRT increases DVT by 300% however, really causes panic and sells papers! Let's look at this in a bit more detail.

If the underlying risk of a DVT (deep venous thrombosis or blood clot in the leg) without HRT is 1 in 10,000 and HRT increases this risk to 3 per 10,000, this would still be considered low risk. However, the tabloids will report this as, "HRT increases risk by 300%!"

The media are not the only people with vested interests.

A colleague of ours recently reported concern that some of the world's menopause societies could be in receipt of funds from the pharmaceutical industry – usually drug companies which produce the hormones.

However, such concerns are surpassed by the anti-HRT lobby who have had press releases in advance of the release of research publications. Their work depends on inducing panic amongst the general public, GPs (particularly) and the government. When you last gave money to cancer research, did you think you were contributing to hundreds of thousands of pounds on inadequate research, using questionnaires in badly designed studies? When we give money to cancer research, we assume the money is to be used for kosher research looking at why cells develop into cancer and how we can treat it – not questionnaires! The only convincing thing about one study was its title – 'The Million Women Study'. A very impressive title but, not only was the study considered by many to be relatively poorly designed, it didn't even have data for a million women!

We do feel generally that research into HRT should be conducted by teams who are regularly involved in managing patients with menopausal symptoms using hormonal treatment.

At this point, you may not be sure whether we are for HRT or against it.

This is our current opinion:

For healthy women below the age of 60, HRT is associated with more benefits than risks. As women get older, delivery through the skin (rather than orally) and the lowest dose, which controls symptoms, is recommended. There is no point at which women must stop treatment – this should be based on an ongoing individualised risk assessment. One of our HRT patients is 83. We will now consider in detail what is known about the menopause and HRT including so what men need to know.

WHAT IS THE MENOPAUSE?
The end of reproductive life.

The best thing about the menopause, the average age being about 51 years, is that there should be no more periods or PMS. That is unless your partner goes onto HRT with a return to regular bleeding and sometimes PMS! However, it is possible to get around all of this.

Historic teaching stated that the menopause coincided with exhaustion of eggs!! It occurs when all of the two million eggs that a woman originally had when she was in the womb herself finally run out. This is not strictly correct as quite a few eggs remain, but they no longer respond to stimulation from the chemical messages (FSH) from the pituitary gland. Remember that each month, during the time of the menstrual bleed a new egg or follicle starts to develop and produces increasing amounts of oestrogen. When there is sufficient oestrogen, the pituitary reduces the chemical message needed to stimulate this follicle – this is follicle stimulating hormone (FSH) – when there is sufficient oestrogen the pituitary stops stimulating the follicle by cutting off the production of FSH. At the menopause, because the follicles fail to develop and do not produce adequate levels of oestrogen, the pituitary increases the strength of its signal by secreting more and more FSH, but this fails to have any effect on the ovary with no increase in oestrogen secretion. This results in very high levels of FSH, but low levels of oestrogen and is the characteristic hormonal state found in the menopause and measuring these hormones can be used for diagnosis. However, in women over age 45, with menopausal symptoms, a blood test is not normally needed to make the diagnosis. The menopausal transition is the period of time leading up to, during and just after the menopause. Strictly speaking the menopause is when the periods stop, but of course a woman will not know that they have completely stopped without waiting for a while – usually 12 months. Menopause is not the only cause of periods stopping. There are other causes of course – pregnancy being one of them!

The menopause transition can go unnoticed or it can be associated with major problems. Hormonal changes are responsible for many symptoms. Ovulation occurs less frequently and this can result in irregular heavy periods. However, you cannot always be sure that abnormal bleeding is hormonal and so more frequent or heavier periods around the time of menopause should always be investigated to make sure that the bleeding is not due to something like cancer of the uterus or ovary.

In the short term, variable hormone levels or lack of oestrogen can give rise to symptoms. Commonly recognised menopausal symptoms include hot flushes and night sweats. Sleep disruption and anxiety are also common, although less well-recognised. Hot flushes are difficult to describe and they seem to be different in different women. In some, the flush spreads up through the neck and into the face. Most women find this embarrassing, even if it is not noticed by other people, although it is often obvious that a woman is having a flush, because they are frantically fanning themselves!

Hot flushes are due to changes in the blood vessels and blood flow – that is why they are called vasomotor symptoms. They may also be accompanied by palpations (rapid and strong beats of the heart like a panic attack). Panic attacks without palpitations may also occur. Sweats can occur day or night, with or without flushing. At night they may result in the bedclothes being thrown on and off. This may cause sleep problems not just for the woman but for you, her partner, too! This can result in much trouble – arguments, separate beds and both being irritable the next day. Loss of sleep (insomnia) may also occur in women who do not have sweats or flushes.

Vaginal symptoms are common and become progressively more likely as women age post menopause. The most common symptoms are vaginal dryness and pain during sexual intercourse with penetrative sex becoming impossible for some women. This is due to lack of oestrogen, which causes thinning of the skin of the vagina, loss of elasticity and lack of lubrication. Thinning of the tissues on the outside can also cause bleeding during attempts to have sex. The dryness and lack of lubrication can occasionally cause soreness in the male and difficulties with performance in many ways. Like the vagina, the bladder also needs oestrogen and deficiency causes urinary tract symptoms including frequency, burning, infection and incontinence. Women may need to get up to pass urine several times a night in common with men due to enlargement of the prostate gland. You might have started to think that it is getting pretty busy in the bedroom for all the wrong reasons after the menopause, what with flushes, the duvet on and off and both parties up and down to the toilet! There are ways to help with all of this.

Mood swings – we have already said in the PMS section of this book that PMS and menopausal symptoms may overlap. Unfortunately, this is not uncommon. What is not known is whether lack of oestrogen causes the mood disturbance or whether it results from all the other symptoms, particularly the poor sleep pattern. Irritability, mood swings and depression can be associated with the menopause. Women may also complain of difficulty with concentration and memory problems. These may be associated with sleep disturbance, mood change or may be directly due to lack of oestrogen. All of these symptoms respond to hormone replacement in the form of HRT.

Long-term health problems as women age can include heart attacks, strokes and osteoporosis. Bone density is measured with a bone densitometer (DEXA). This is like a mini x-ray of certain parts of the body, usually the hip, spine and, occasionally, the heel.

Tests have shown that up until the age of 30, bone density progressively increases. After 30, bone is lost for the rest of life, so osteoporosis is inevitable eventually. It is a more significant problem for women, because men start with much more bone than women and when the menopause "arrives" there is a further rapid loss of bone. Men also continue to produce their sex hormone (testosterone) until a much later age. The more rapid development of osteoporosis can result in hip fractures (neck of femur, NOF), which can be a threat to life in older woman. Fracture of the forearm is also common in women (dinner fork deformity). Fractures or collapse of the vertebral spine can result in pressure on nerves, loss of height and in advanced cases the typical stoop of a "dowager's hump". All post-menopausal women sustaining a fracture should have a DEXA scan to measure bone density. This will enable treatment to be offered if required.

Remember that there are three hormones, which come from the ovary, oestrogen, progesterone and testosterone (the "male" hormone). Quite a lot of male hormone is produced from the ovary but not as much as in men obviously. After the menopause there is virtually no oestrogen, no progesterone and testosterone levels fall significantly. Testosterone, with oestrogen, is very important for sex drive, because as well as all the problems described above, sex drive may disappear completely.

Vaginal pain, no lubrication, bleeding and no sex drive and men wonder why their partners seem reluctant to have sex after the menopause!

This may be a bit of an exaggeration, but you can see where the tensions come from in a relationship.

WHO "GETS" THE MENOPAUSE?
Well, all women "get the menopause" eventually, but not necessarily the symptoms. Most women get symptoms (say about 75%), although only about 10–15% will seek treatment from their doctor.

The average age of the menopause is 51 and it is normal to reach the menopause between the ages of 45 and 55. Below 45 is early, but not considered premature. Below age 40, the menopause is considered abnormal and this is called premature ovarian insufficiency.

Professor Shaughn O'Brien & Dr Paula Briggs

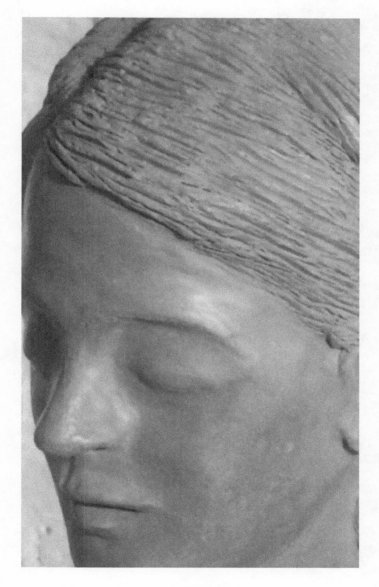

Menopause Solved 2015

HerHormones

CHAPTER 12

Treatment of the Menopause

Can hormones be avoided?

What hormone treatment is there?

What are the long term effects?

What are the benefits of treatment?

What are the risks of treatment?

Can the Menopause be treated without hormones and can your partner avoid doctors?

The simple answer is yes. However, as the problem is due to lack of oestrogen, the most effective treatment is oestrogen, although many women are keen to avoid oestrogen and in this case it is worth exploring alternatives. But beware, there are many charlatans out there trying to "flog" unproven treatments!

Most of these treatment options can be bought from "health food" shops. Actually, they are often much more expensive than prescription drugs and the main reason that they have not been shown to be associated with a higher incidence of breast cancer (particularly the "natural" plant oestrogens) is because no proper studies have ever been done!

But conventional medicine and doctors can be avoided which must be good even if alternative remedies do not work!

There are several non-hormonal drugs, which can be used for treating menopausal symptoms, but they are largely ineffective. One drug called venlafaxine has been shown in a couple of studies to improve hot flushes. It is technically an antidepressant (a bit like Prozac), and some women benefit from a reduction in flushes (and probably an improvement their mood disorder if they have one).

Clonidine has a licence to treat hot flushes, but it is rarely effective.

Newer drugs (NK antagonist drugs), which were originally developed to treat alcoholism are being investigated in early stage clinical trials and may in future offer treatment for breast cancer survivors.

The best way of managing menopausal symptoms is by replacing what the woman is deficient in – oestrogen. This results in well documented, consistent symptom control.

There are many different ways in which oestrogen can be given.

Some preparations put the levels of hormone in the blood stream back up to normal – others act only where they are put. That essentially means that they are put in the vagina to have a local effect on the vagina and bladder without going into the blood stream and we will come back to these later.

If we wish to return the hormone levels in the blood stream to normal treatment can be given as follows:

Tablets: This is the most widely used approach. A drug called Premarin has been given to many women. This is conjugated equine oestrogens which, translated, is "a mixture of horse oestrogens". These have been sold as being natural – extracted from horse's urine and not synthesised in the laboratory. Some women do not like the idea of this either because of the thought of horse urine or because they are vegetarian or because they are concerned about animal rights. Allegedly some of the drug companies that make synthetic oestrogen employed PR companies to place pictures of decrepit looking horses with urine catheters and bags attached in order to boost sales of the synthetic variety! This is apocryphal.

So oral treatment may be with conjugated equine oestrogens or the synthetic variety (which is nearer to the body's natural oestrogen – synthetic but more natural – isn't life confusing!). Tablets are taken every day. Remember in the normal spontaneous hormone cycle we said that the ovary produces progesterone in the second half of the cycle. A progestogen is included in the pack of sequential HRT and this reflects the predictability of the menstrual cycle and it also prevents cancer of the lining of the womb, by preventing overstimulation with oestrogen. This is very important and if you have gone straight to this chapter without looking at Chapters 1 and 2, you are advised to go back to the beginning!

For this reason, a usual HRT pack will contain one tablet, which is taken every day (oestrogen) and a different one which is taken for about 12–14 days (oestrogen and progestogen). Because the tablets recreate the hormone cycle comparable to that of a premenopausal woman, the lining of the uterus builds up and sheds just like it does in a normal cycle. The downside to this type of regime is that "periods" return, but they tend to be lighter and more predictable.

There are some combinations, which have oestrogen and progestogen every day, without there being a cycle. With these, although there is no cycle unfortunately there can sometimes be unexpected bleeding, which would need to be investigated. This usually occurs if this type of hormone treatment is commenced too soon after a woman has her last period. The recommended gap is 12 months or around age 54 if she is already taking the type of tablet associated with a regular bleed.

There is yet another HRT preparation called tibolone, taken by mouth which does much the same, using a single hormone which has the same effects as oestrogen, progesterone and testosterone – tibolone

The other delivery routes used for HRT are, transdermal (patches, gels and a spray), subdermal (implants) and vaginal preparations.

Many women and health experts continue to struggle with HRT since the turnaround in attitude toward hormone therapy in the wake of the Women's Health Initiative (WHI) trial. This was designed to investigate the effect on long term health associated with the use of combined oestrogen and progestogen (conjugated equine oestrogen and medroxyprogesterone acetate). The trial was stopped early, in 2002, because hormone users were found to have a higher risk of breast cancer, heart disease, strokes, and blood clots. Although the added risks were small, many women and their clinicians concluded that they must discontinue hormone therapy. Countless women found that hot flushes, sleep disturbance, and other menopausal symptoms returned with a vengeance.

Hormone therapy is still considered the most effective treatment for menopausal symptoms. NICE Guidance published in November 2015 and updated in December 2019 and new media interest on the beneficial effects of HRT are slowly repairing the damage done by the press coverage of the WHI study. Between 2002 and 2015 there was no research or education in relation to menopause. During that time, one concern of health experts was that women were turning to alternatives that they thought were safer, but this may not have been the case.

Even before the WHI results came in, many women were looking for something different to relieve hot flushes, night sweats and vaginal dryness. Some women disliked the side effects of hormone therapy, such as breast tenderness or the reintroduction of regular or irregular bleeding. Others worried about the potential link of oestrogen with breast cancer. Then there were women opposed to taking drugs for symptoms because doing so implies that menopause is a disease rather than a normal part of life. Others objected to the use of pregnant mares' urine — the source of oestrogen in oral conjugated equine oestrogens (Premarin) described above and the only oestrogen tested in the WHI trial.

IN SEARCH OF "NATURAL" REMEDIES
Many women assume that "natural" hormones are better or safer — but the term "natural" is open to interpretation.

Any product for which the principal ingredient has an animal, plant, or mineral source is technically natural. It doesn't matter whether the substance is ground, put into capsules, and sold over the counter — or extracted in a laboratory, manufactured by a pharmaceutical company, and made available only by prescription. For example, the soy plant is the source of supplements that some women take to ease menopausal symptoms; it is also used, along with yams, to make the oestrogen in the FDA-approved hormone drug Estrace.

But unlike Estrace, soy supplements which can be bought over the counter aren't regulated and haven't been rigorously tested in humans, so we don't know whether they're safe or effective. There is some evidence that certain soy components may actually stimulate breast tumour growth. So "natural" doesn't necessarily equal "safe" — and may simply be a euphemism for "unregulated".

"Bioidentical" hormone therapy should not to be confused with "body identical" hormone therapy available on prescription. Both resemble naturally occurring hormones in structure but the compounded hormones are provided by specialist pharmacies or whereas the body identical hormones are regulated and developed in the conventional way, authorised by regulators such as the Medicines and Healthcare products Regulatory Agency (MHRA).

Regulated body identical hormones act in the body just like the hormones we produce ourselves and they are the most like naturally occurring hormones. But here again, that tricky word *natural* muddies the waters. Pregnant mares' urine is natural, but Premarin is not body identical, at least not compared to human oestrogen.

Are body identical hormones safer? Yes, if oestradiol is delivered through the skin as a patch or a gel it does not increase the risk of blood clots in the leg or lung over and above the individual woman's inherent risk. Blood clots like this are the commonest significant side effect associated with use of HRT. Women taking body identical oestrogen who have a uterus must still take a progestogen or micronised progesterone (body identical) to prevent endometrial cancer.

CURRENT RECOMMENDATIONS FOR HORMONE REPLACEMENT THERAPY

The current advice in the UK for women using HRT, in consultation with their GP and/or gynaecologist, is to use the lowest dose which provides symptom control, for the shortest period of time. Given the findings from new research, the risks associated with the use of HRT are low and duration of use may, if necessary, be extended, as the use of HRT for many women provides welcome relief from distressing postmenopausal symptoms. Based on the current evidence, starting HRT at the early onset of the menopause, and carrying on for a few years carries little risk in healthy women. All women commencing HRT should be advised of type, dose, mode of delivery and duration, and doctors should tailor treatment to individual patients.

HOT OFF THE PRESS

It has taken us some years to write this book and as we finish this penultimate chapter, new treatments are appearing in the research and lay press on a daily basis. So at least the delay in completing the book means that you are reading the latest material!

LASER THERAPY FOR THE VULVA AND VAGINA

For women who do not wish to or are not allowed to use oestrogen (e.g. a breast cancer patient) there are now new ways to treat vaginal atrophy. Whilst the standard method is to use oestrogen locally as pessaries, cream, gel or an impregnated ring, an alternative to this is to use this new technique. Both CO_2 and erbium YAG laser cause minimal discomfort and regenerate collagen, improving tissue quality. More research is needed to determine the number of treatments applied. Current recommendations are for women to have three treatments initially and an additional treatment once a year. However, women who have had breast cancer may need more treatments initially in order to optimise the beneficial effects. These are evident in most women for the external genitalia, the vagina and also the bladder. At present these treatments are not available on the NHS and are costly in the region of £700 per treatment. However, women are willing to spend money on many cosmetic procedures and this one has definite benefits for men as well!

OVARIAN TRANSPLANTATION

If ovarian tissue is removed at keyhole surgery and the acquired tissue is preserved by freezing, this can be re-implanted into another part of the body at a later stage so that ovarian function – ovulation and hormone production – can be recommenced, possibly many years down the line. This has been developed mainly for patients who are about to experience a premature menopause due to the drugs or radiation-induced in cancer therapy. These patients develop a chemical or radiation menopause and are thus prematurely menopausal and infertile. When the patient has completed therapy and is well, she can have the tissue re-implanted and hormones relieve the menopause and ovulation from the tissue recommences permitting a potential pregnancy. This has already been undertaken with success and is a very major step forward.

Of course, it is also possible that preserved tissue can be re-implanted at the age of the natural menopause and then the menopause, its symptoms and risks delayed for many years. This is the angle the media have taken recently and was not the original intention, but watch this space!

For further information on the Menopause see:
British Menopause Society www.thebms.org.uk
Menopause Matters www.menopausematters.co.uk
Premature Menopause www.daisy@daisynetwork.org.uk

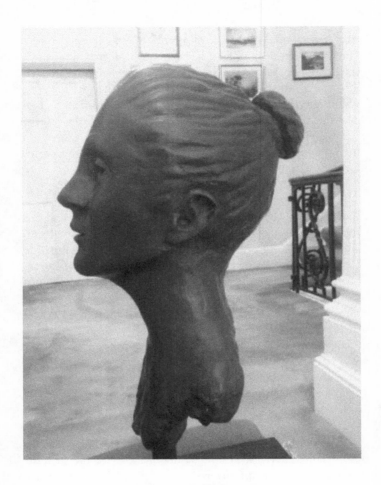

Portrait of a Young Woman 2015

Professor Shaughn O'Brien & Dr Paula Briggs

HerHormones

CHAPTER 13

An anecdote!

This 'chapter' is dedicated to a good friend of one of the authors who frequently offers to swap jobs for the day. PMSOB would get to be a managing director as a mechanical engineer in the car industry for a day, and he would be a gynaecologist for the day. His salary would be attractive!

For his 60th he was given a very convincing mock Voucher for a Day's Job Swap, he as a gynaecologist, together with the required equipment! We have never been quite sure whether he believed it or not – he did make a big reference to it in his after-dinner speech. He was finally persuaded not to show the audience the speculum during his speech from his "present pack".

I only include this little anecdote because as this is a book for men it may be appreciated by you and because the story is totally true.

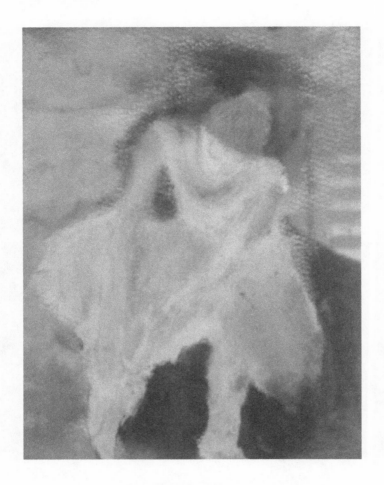

The Young Dancer 2008

CHAPTER 14

Evolutionary benefit?

MERE SPECULATION BUT POSSIBLY TRUE...MENSTRUATION

There is unlikely to be any evolutionary advantage associated with menstruation; as we demonstrated earlier, menstruation is a function of modern life with limited pregnancies and fertility control.

MENOPAUSE

There can of course be no evolutionary advantage associated with the menopause because by definition it occurs after reproductive life has ceased. It may have a role in the nurturing of our children's children: grandchildren. But again the menopause is a modern phenomenon – in the distant past, the average woman died around the same age as the menopause.

Surely painful periods, endometriosis, PCOS and subfertility cannot offer any species survival benefit, but may be PMS does? We have considered this in a "tongue in cheek" fashion, but maybe there is a credibility to this theory. Assume that sexual intercourse does not occur for the first five days of the cycle because of menstruation. This of course is not universally true, but many women /men/couples find sex whilst bleeding aesthetically distasteful or taboo and many religions forbid it.

Sexual desire is influenced positively by oestrogen and testosterone, both of which are produced by the ovaries. Oestrogen reaches its peak by the 13th or 14th day of the cycle which, probably not coincidentally, is the point in time where the follicle containing the egg (ovum) is ready to be released and the lining of the uterus is well prepared to receive the fertilised egg, if fertilisation actually occurs. Remember the other effect of the hormonal variation in the cycle is the change in the mucus in the cervix. When the oestrogen levels are high, the cervical mucus becomes thin and watery so that the sperm pass freely through into the uterus. How convenient then, when everything is just right the female becomes sociable and sexually receptive! Well, either this is by design if you are a creationist or bred into the human species if you believe Darwin. When ovulation has occurred, there is no longer any "biological" purpose for sex. Indeed, there may be benefits of not having sperm reaching an egg which is "older" as it is possible that miscarriage or fetal abnormality may be more common.

So what happens after ovulation? Well firstly, in response to the increasing levels of progesterone, the cervical mucus becomes thick and the sperm cannot penetrate it even if sex does occur. Secondly and (of particular importance to the issues in the earlier chapter on PMS) progesterone has a negative effect on the mood and sociability of women once ovulation has occurred. Millennia ago, when it was advantageous to increase population numbers, sexual activity would have been promoted by the female around the time of ovulation, but in the days/weeks after ovulation, men would be frightened off by the aggressive antisocial female. Males in primitive society would avoid the premenstrual female and seek more sociable, receptive *ovulating* women. So, maybe negative physiological premenstrual symptoms are a normal physiological part of the menstrual cycle, built in for evolutionary benefit. But not for 20th Century women!!!

Evidently, the male seeking ovulating females is also of evolutionary benefit and so is polygamy in males the norm? Doesn't account for affairs in menopausal women!! Or maybe that is sexual liberation, when fear of pregnancy no longer exists!? This may be countered by the fact that as the menopause approaches levels of hormones, both testosterone and oestrogen diminish, with virtually no oestrogen and low testosterone post menopause. Libido in all women declines, mostly slowly but sometimes abruptly around the menopause. Talking purely biologically again there are no eggs being produced and so there is no real purpose in sex (apart from pleasure!). Even then, that can be affected by the impact of oestrogen deficiency on the urogenital tissues (vulva, vagina and bladder). In men, in comparison to women, the decline in libido is much more gradual and the sperm count remains high into old age – so the male menopause and the desire to have a sports car and a younger woman is perhaps explained by evolution!

MORE ANECDOTES
It is well known that hormones can influence the human voice. The pill changes the pitch of women's voices. When male hormones are given to women, their voices can become slightly deeper and huskier.

Danazol is a drug that was used to treat endometriosis in the past (see chapter 10); it was associated with some male side effects, including an alteration of pitch and timbre of the woman's voice. A guitarist and folk singer was once treated for endometriosis. She came back with no endometriosis, and delighted that her voice had gone down a semitone and she said, when singing, it had become much sexier!

Another patient (not one of ours) who was a high-flying opera soprano dropped her voice significantly, so that she could no longer sing soprano and she was not at all pleased! The menopause and the menstrual cycle can have a deleterious effect on the singing voice. Maria Callas (a famous operatic soprano in the first half of 20th century) experienced significant deterioration of her voice as she became perimenopausal. She was dropping notes at a recording session and blamed her menstrual cycle, having obviously noticed the link. The fact that she was well past menopause suggests that the loss of pitch, quality, timbre and overtones was associated with lack of oestrogen and a small number of research studies have since demonstrated this. So it is possible (back to evolution at last) that a combination of deepening, thinning or shrillness of the voice could be off putting, with men consequently seeking the more soothing oestrogenised tone and quality of the voice that they find in younger women.

PHEROMONES
Linked to the factors relating sexual attractiveness to hormones, is the possible connection associated with pheromones.

What are pheromones?
Well firstly there are a lot of them about. A lot is known about some, virtually nothing is known about others.

They produce a "smell" sometimes obvious, like musk and at other times not obviously detectable with the *smell* the equivalent of a high-pitched dog whistle, that cannot be heard by humans. Some of the simplest insects produce pheromones as part of their active reproductive cycle. Many animals do too, and a "positive pheromone attraction" may occur in relation to the high oestrogen phase of the menstrual cycle leading up to ovulation. It may initially seem unlikely that the smell of the female human causes sexual attraction – but why not? Women possibly produce attractive pheromones in response to oestrogen production leading up to ovulation and then post ovulation it is equally possible that unattractive pheromones are produced. Even Jo Malone can't fix that!! In modern society, the attraction between the sexes is no longer solely for the purpose of producing offspring to expand the population, and women will wish to be attractive to males at all times of the month. Is this the original reason women began to use perfume - to mask the smell of the unattractive premenstrual pheromones?

We also wondered if there could be an effect of male pheromones on the female?

Well obviously there is no menstrual cycle for the male. But let's assume that males produce the same pheromone all of the time. Let's also assume that women can smell this pheromone. It is well known that some women find the smell of musk-like pheromones attractive – manly and sexual. Others find it offensive, comparable to smelly armpits! We are fairly sure that no one has ever done an experiment where women's perception of pheromones has been tested in individual women at different phases of the menstrual cycle. Female sense of smell almost certainly changes through the cycle and so the same pheromone released by the male partner can cause different responses in the female at different times in her menstrual cycle – at ovulation she perceives it as sexy and attractive, but after ovulation, overpowering and repulsive. She may also find you repulsive generally at different phases of the menstrual cycle – so things are not going well for anyone in the week or so leading up to menstruation, and that can be incredibly confusing when you become the object of her sexual desire not so many days later around the time of ovulation!

Natural family planning and methods of contraception "abusing" the science behind them are particularly confusing for women (and disappointing). When you most feel like sex, don't do it!!!! You might get pregnant but if we go back to evolution, the only reason for sex is to achieve a pregnancy. Thank God for the pill and for specific hormonal combinations for women with PMS, to both treat the condition and provide contraception. The optimal way of ensuring that sexuality is preserved in otherwise healthy women post menopause is to ensure access to oestrogen (to manage a deficiency state in women who would have been dead in a previous era), progestogen (to protect the lining of the womb) and testosterone (to protect sexual desire). There has been no "proper" research (in a systematic way) as far as we know, but this is something that individual couples can explore, until some scientist decides it is important enough to research – a behavioural research psychologist could easily turn this into a PhD! A little anecdote to conclude our book. A woman, a florist, was sat next to her gynaecologist at a dinner and they got around to talking about jobs, children and hormones as one does. She had finished having children by the age of 22. Now in her early forties, with her children off to university, she had a feeling of lack of purpose although she was nowhere near the menopause. It may be that for the many women who have completed their families by their early twenties or thirties, blaming hormones and the end of reproductive capacity is not correct. The way they feel at this stage is due purely to children leaving "the nest" rather than the influence of hormones.

Important message to women: Do not blame hormones for everything – other things may coincide in time with physiological changes and that does not necessarily mean that one causes the other.

Important message to men: A great degree of change occurs both premenstrually and around the time of the menopause. This can be very challenging and frequently leads women to question their self-worth.

A combination of tolerance, sensitivity and increased attention is required by you. We hope that this small book will help you to do that by better understanding how hormones affect women and indirectly men.

Professor Shaughn O'Brien & Dr Paula Briggs

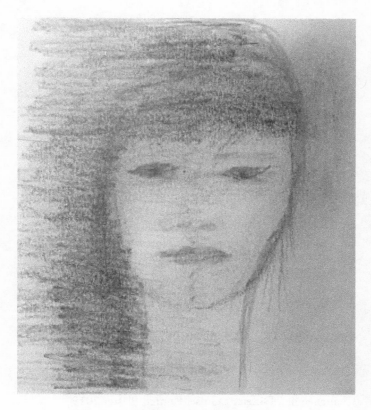

Preliminary Sketch of a Young Women 2018

List of Illustrations

Professor Shaughn O'Brien & Dr Paula Briggs

Study for Portrait, Print 2019

Sketch for Portrait of a Young Woman 2018

Figure of a Young Woman, Jesmonite 2019

Figures 1 – 13 Hand drawn as would be used in a consultation and explanation to patients

All illustration of sculptures, sketches, prints, graphs and images are

Contact: shrewsburyartscub@hotmail.com

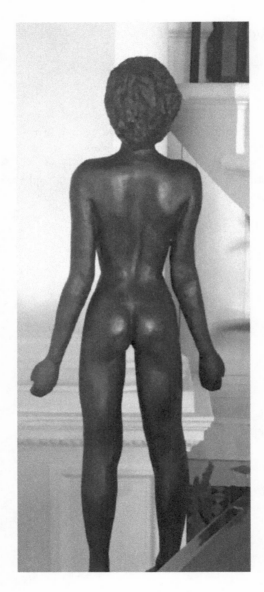

Figure of a young woman 2019

Professor Shaughn O'Brien & Dr Paula Briggs

Afterword

The contents of this book are *not* intended to replace advice from medical professionals. We advise readers to consult an appropriate medical practitioner if necessary.

9 781913 568153